Life Force Press
*

Tai Chi Diet
Ch'ang Ming

(REVISED BOOK)
was Tai Chi Diet: food for life.

Written by
Professor Myke Symonds©Copyright-2008 & 2021

All rights reserved Internationally

No parts of this publication may be reproduced, stored in a retrieval system,
copied or transmitted in any form or by any means, electronic, mechanical,
photocopying, recording, manually or otherwise without the prior permission of
the author copyright owner.

British Library Cataloguing In Publication Data
A Record of this Publication is available
from the British Library

ISBN: 9780954293239

First Published in Paperback
2007 by
Life Force Publishing
This Revised Edition 2021

www.Life-Force-Publishing.co.uk

-o-

OTHER BOOKS BY THE AUTHOR OR COMING SOON

These are the main books planned within the Practical Taoist range of books from Life Force Books, an offshoot of the Heaven & Earth Way Academy of Chinese Taoist Arts (www.tttkungfu.com), otherwise known as The Way of Heaven & Earth School, or Tiandidao (Modern Romanised) or T'ien Ti Tao (Trad. Romanised Chinese).

Practical Philosophy of Tao (2nd Edition)
The Way of Nature - an Easy Learning Guide.
Description: The Taoists for thousands of years have learned to work in harmony with Nature. The basic philosophic principles entwine through exercise, medicine, diet, self-defence systems and much more. This is the first time a book has been written in plain English that uncovers the mysticism. From food to sex and relationships, the relativity of Tao makes sense.

Tai Chi Diet: (this book, previously POD via Five Elements)
Description: For many centuries the Chinese Taoists have known the secrets of balanced diet and good health. Foods are like medicine or poison, such as herbs (another form of food), they can heal or make ill. Learn how to detect illness or imbalance, how to correct your diet and live longer with more energy. Special needs section covers common illnesses like cancer, migraines, hypoglycaemia, rheumatism and more.

Qi-gong & Baduanjin.
Description: Gentle breathing and stretching for resilient health and healing. Qi-gong is deceptively simple yet amazingly effective. It has been used in China to cure cancer, perform operations without drugs (anaesthetics) and to help common illnesses such as rheumatism and hypertension, heart, lung and digestive problems. In this book we look at some common imbalances and the correct qi-gong approach for each.

Life Force – Taoist Kung-fu
Practical Taoist Kung-fu, also known as 'Wudang Kung-fu', is not just about fighting, although very effective. In Taoist Kung-fu we learn how to 'balance' exercises so that we lessen risk of injury, gain flexibility and improve health and strength in a more natural manner. The techniques taught are all practical but at the same time very adaptable, thus giving the long-term practitioner a superb arsenal with which to protect himself with. The long-term health benefits are enormous too, physically and mentally.

Tao & Taoism - A Practical Philosophy (to come)

Taoist 'Open Gate' Yoga (to come)

Others may follow.

Life Force Publishing:
www.Life-Force-Publishing.com

DEDICATIONS AND SINCERE THANKS

Dedicated to all those who suffer needlessly.

Thanks to Lou Lloyd & Terry Windsor

for Proofing & Suggestions

*

WITH SINCERE THANKS AND GRATITUDE TO:

The Late Grandmaster C. Chee Soo

All the "Tao Science" Developers, past and present.

My students and friends for their encouragement.

*

The Taoist Arts are not about personal gain,

Although we have to live.

The Arts concern the quality of life,

And when we learn we give.

*

"T'ai Chi Diet" is the Author's nickname for Ch'ang Ming (Long Life) Diet, which began many centuries ago in the Wu Tang or Wudang Mountains in China. Home to many Taoist study centres. T'ai Chi Ch'uan is the exercise-come-self-defence Art which is fashioned on the philosophy of Tao, and it means "Supreme Ultimate" and/or Universe. The Universe is the Supreme Ultimate and can never never be reshaped or beaten. Likewise, the T'ai Chi Diet is the only diet that will ever make sense to human life.

CONTENTS
INGREDIENTS

Introduction	Page 06
The Balanced Power -	
Overview of Taoist principles	Page 09
Chinese Names Pronunciation Guide	Page 13
Tao Science - The Supreme Ultimate	Page 14
Universal Observations	Page 17
Six Part Health Tests	Page 25
The Yin/Yang of Body Language	Page 40
Let's face It	Page 40
Symptoms & Illnesses	Page 45
TCM Diagnostic Principles	Page 50
Food & Exercise	Page 61

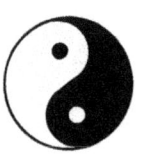

Preparation	**Page 67**
Yin/Yang Foods	Page 69
General Advice	Page 70
Five Rules for Healthier Eating	Page 71
Taoist Dietary Guidelines	Page 74
What This Book Is All About!	**Page 76**
Yin/Yang Table of Foods	Page 78
Detox Plan	Page 80
Meat or Veg? Doctor's Independent Review	Page 83
The Five Elements	Page 87
Case Histories	Page 91
Five Element Theory Table	Page 95

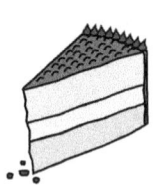

Basic Food Properties	**Page 96**
Minerals & Their Function	Page 98
Daily Vitamin & Mineral Needs	Page 103
Vitamins and their functions	Page 105
Vitamin Vital Statistics	Page 106

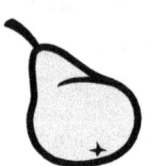

Minerals and their functions	Page 111
Tips For Eating & Better Health	Page 117
Baby Foods	Page 118
Hyperactivity in Children	Page 120
Fats	Page 120
Nutritional Advice For All	Page 122
Nutrition - the value of food	Page 124
Nutritional Building Blocks	Page 127

LET'S GET COOKING!
Foods With Attitude! — **Page 133**

The good, the bad and the ugly:

The Ginseng Hunters	Page 144
Elderberry	Page 150
Making Changes	Page 154
List and Lose	Page 158

Special Needs Section — **Page 163**

Arthritis - Rheumatism, etc.	Page 165
Cancer (Tumours)	Page 173
Hypoglycaemia (Low Blood Sugar)	Page 184
Hyperglycaemia	Page 190
Irritable Bowel Syndrome	Page 193
VIRUS – Corona (Covid) or other.	Page 199

A Sensible Diet - What is it today? — **Page 215**

Dietetics, Herbs, Drugs or What?	Page 218
Supplements	Page 223
Complimentary Exercises	Page 225
The author's background and other information.	Page 228
Bibliography	Page 230

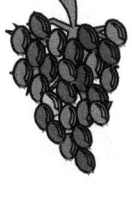

INTRODUCTION

As a child born after World War 2, I grew up in a period where food was rationed and most families had to get by on a marginal diet. We had very few treats, unlike the kids of today who seem to live on treats alone. The best treats I had were after our Bramley apple tree had produced its wonderful bitter-sweet crop and my mother had made home cooked apple pies or apple fritters from them. Delicious was hardly a good enough word to describe them. On Xmas morning I would awake and make my way down to the kitchen. There hanging over the fireplace were two Xmas Stockings (Large Red Socks, basically) with our special treats in them. One treat was a fresh orange. Yes, an Orange. What an alien luxury!
    Life was not easy for parents in those times and diets were often lacking; constipation was a frequent problem, caused usually by too many eggs in our diets as these became more readily available after the war.

There are now, in the 21st Century, far more types of foods available to every type of cook and individual. People from the Caribbean can buy Caribbean fruit and vegetables, even though they are in a different climate where not so warm and sunny, so foodstuffs are imported by air or sea. Even though the Supermarkets are packed full of exotic foods, trying to choose the healthiest options may not always be as straightforward as we may think. We can now get food from all over the world; apples and Kiwi fruit from New Zealand, tomatoes and other fruits from Spain or Italy, grains from China or America and varied oddments from Brazil or Mexico. But is this good? In some cases yes, in some cases no - you will have to read the book to find out!

Many people suffer common maladies that are generally accepted by our society as 'normal' illnesses. There is no such thing as a *normal* illness, for all illness is an imbalance that has been caused by 'tilting the scales' (in this case of our diet) too far one way. Correcting this imbalance may require leaving that particular food which caused the 'sway out' of our diet and counteracting it with something else to get back on course. In terms of health and illness, proper balance is *normal* and anything outside of that is abnormal and therefore should be eradicated and corrected. Sages of the East observed health matters over thousands of years and learned many things. This book blends the essential ingredients of Eastern Macrobiotic Dietary Principles, Taoist philosophy and general nutritional information for a longer, healthier lifestyle which, if followed and adhered to, can eliminate many of the unpleasant illnesses from your life and enable you to liberate yourself to far happier dimensions in work, play, relationships and social positions.

The Taoists of Wu Tang/Wudang in central China, have been studying health and healing and beneficial exercise since the Wu Tang Mountain retreats (called Temples by those who don't know!) were first built. The subject goes back way further than that, right back to a very scholarly gentleman called Huang Ti – The first Emperor of China who was nicknamed 'The Yellow Emperor', Born 2711 BCE and Died 2598 BCE (aged 113 years.)

My own personal background is wide and long. After studying many Eastern philosophies and beliefs, I am essentially a Taoist: which means I Study Tao, the *Natural* Universal Way, or just "Way" but referring to the Way of Nature. Since mid-to-late childhood I have studied psychology, sociology and observed the way that humans interact, what causes issues and what resolves issues. Jobs have been varied, covering many aspects of life, which has given me opportunity to meet many interesting people and observe even more. Not all roses, as they say, as I have been victimised by people who are sick of mind and unbalanced, on several occasions. You try to help some people and they *transfer* their psychological problems on to you, just because you are an easy target. That must never stop you from progressing though. If you wish to help others, then first you must help yourself, or heal yourself if your lifestyle is imbalanced.

By studying this book you will be able to gain thousands of years worth of knowledge and apply it wisely to your own life. In writing these books for you I hope that you will become a master of your own life, as much as Tao allows, and in return for my efforts to help you I pass on that commitment to you to help at least ten others liberate themselves from sickness and imbalance, be it physical, mental or spiritual, and in turn you may pass on this same commitment to them.

May the 'Life Force' be with you.

Prof. Myke Symonds (Author) Instructor for 48 years and Student of life since childhood. Has studied diet and the effects of food, philosophy, psychology, social behaviour, plus mainstream Eastern belief systems, T'ai Chi Ch'uan, Tao Ch'uan-shu, Ch'i Kung, TCM and Lay healing: all part of a Holistic Taoist lifestyle and school.

THE BALANCED POWER
Overview of Taoist principles.

This book was first started in 1982, available then only as a rough guide to students and friends until 2007. Inspired by the Chinese Taoist Macrobiotic Diet, nicknamed Ch'ang Ming or Zhang ming (meaning "Long Life", or alternatively Macrobiotic from the Greek 'Macros' = Great or Long, and 'Bios' = Life) as taught to me by my old Taoist Arts Master, Professor Clifford Chee Soo and also previously inspired by George Oshawa. The macrobiotic diet is not a fad or weight-loss gimmick but deals with the *balance* of foods. Yin foods may contain (among other elements) potassium, whilst Yang foods may contain sodium – salt is very high in sodium. The body is made up of the chemicals, minerals and vitamins we consume combined with the fluids we drink. Therefore it should be plain to see that addressing the issues of imbalance should help restore balance leading to better health. There were a couple of expressions I heard somewhere years ago which I think sums up the way most people treat their bodies: "If you put contaminated fuel in your car then you would not be surprised if it broke down and even died on you", and "Most people treat their cars better than their bodies!"

Tao (pronounced 'Tao' in Central and Northern China and 'Dow' in Southern China) refers to the Forces of the Universe and everything that happens naturally and hence means 'The Way'. Taoism is *not* a religion, it is a philosophy relating to simple everyday life sciences, the WAY of LIVING. If anyone want to wear beads or chant Mantras to remind themselves what they are doing, then that's their business. Translation from Chinese to English is somewhat ambiguous and one has to take into consideration the context of many other parts of the sentence or conversation in which the word is used. In this instance we can broaden the sense of the word 'Way' into something like this; 'Universal Power that has no fixed form but forms everything within our Universe, known or not, seen or not, felt or not.' Shall we call it Nature's 'Life Force' for the sake of saving our breath and/or my fingers?

If we do not view things from a correct perspective our vista may be tainted by preconceptions (education and previous beliefs) which are biased to our limited daily needs within an industrialised society. European culture is oldest towards the Mediterranean area and India. Indian and Oriental culture goes back thousands of years further still; in China there was a highly civilised culture around five thousand years ago. In Great Britain men and women were extremely primitive around two-thousand years ago, just before the Romans invaded. The Americas, as we think of them today, are even younger, although there were tribes of Native Americans who had their own particular 'natural' cultures. Chinese inventions range from the first mechanical clock, typewriter, banknotes, paper making, compass, gunpowder (including mortars, bombs and rockets) to iron founding, bridge building, irrigation, surgery (using bamboo acupuncture needles in heart swapping surgery; two-hundred years before Christ!) and even the common wheelbarrow were all Chinese firsts, to name but a few. The Chinese discovered the world in 1421.

Considering the British arrogance between the 1700's and 1900's, it was hardly surprising that those who came from the West to bring their 'fabulous new culture to the savages' (usually diseases and unfair trading) were known as Gweilos or 'White Foreign Devils' among some Chinese (this was because the men used to wear white wigs and powder their faces to be white). Had it not have been for such phenomenal Western cock-ups like the Tea and Opium Wars there would have been far better relationships far sooner and in the UK life would be better now, probably, bar the odd dictator or two. The outstanding store of knowledge within the Chinese culture then could have married with our own medical developments to produce a much better modern health care service. At least we have the intelligence these days to communicate with some other cultures. It is only now that we are [slowly] discovering the wonders of all the accumulated medical wealth in the word, particularly China [this was written in the 1980's, but China seems to be going the same way as the West now, downhill with Orthodox Medicines and Drugs].

Many influences were brought to bear upon the development of Chinese Arts, with Confucius, Taoist and Buddhist influences being the main ones. Generally though, I would say that it is still the collective 'Chinese Mind' that is the most marked and remarkable. Obviously a few people stood out from the crowd, like 'The Yellow Emperor' Huang Ti and Lao Tzu or (Doctor) Hua T'o, the man who invented Acupuncture. These people inspired many thousands of others to take up the cause to find better ways of living in harmony with Nature's Life Force and in doing so gathered the principles together which describe these forces. Thus TAO became the term for all things in harmony with Nature and it was easily recognised that if we are a product of Nature then anything we do which is 'unnatural' can be corrected by using a 'natural' remedial method.

It is a human folly to use the potentially powerful mind that we have to destroy ourselves by experimenting with 'artificial' inventions; this includes synthesised and altered food, powerfully dangerous drugs and vaccines. The Taoist overview is not one of religious zest, nor personal gain; it is that of a holistic and 'green' view of the natural laws of the Universe. In our Universe only that which is natural survives intact or transmutes in a healthy and perfectly normal manner. Things that are man made tend to go wrong at some point; probably due to imbalances in the structural harmonies, which cause other imbalances as a by-product. There are some things that cannot be bettered and should not be tampered with - the food we eat is one example. Take another example, the human egg: The egg, produced in the females' ovaries, is naturally formed from the Mother's tissues and the quality of the egg cell may be influenced by what she eats, drinks or otherwise puts into her body. The genes that determine the baby's gender and growth peculiarities may also be affected by past generations and their own formations, so deficient diets or other developmental factors can produce damaged genes which may be passed on from one generation to another, unless corrected, which may also take a long time to repair. Western medical tests carried out in the 1970's suggested that men who smoke cannabis or drink too much alcohol (both Yin after-effects) are more likely to produce sperm which will likely result in female babies rather than male. The most likely chance of producing male babies normally lies with the wife's side of the family; if her mother and grandmother produced more boys than girls then the likelihood of a boy child was increased. This theory has for hundreds of years gone beyond drugs.

The Chinese knew about the effects of what we put into our body and have a name for the resulting dietary recommendations, 'Zhang ming (Ch'ang Ming)' - Long Life diet. The Taoist influences were again the greatest here. If it were not for the studies of many Taoists the Balanced Power of Life would never have been observed and many, many more thousands of people worldwide would be prematurely dead. Unfortunately, although I have always been keen to find out more, I have not been so enthused about keeping records. Hence, there is little bibliography to go with this book. Suffice it to say that over the course of the years I have come across many interesting facts and study results that deserved to be noted. However, the real use of these facts lies in their adoption, not recording. As you know, it is one thing to talk about a subject and another to take it on board and actuate it.

Every great journey of 1,000 miles begins with just one step.

So goes the ancient Chinese saying. Keep this in mind throughout the reading of this book. You will come to a section that suggests you "list and lose". In essence it states that you should find just one thing, to begin with, in your diet with which you are not happy, or now recognise you need to change because of its *ill* effects. Replace one thing and get used to it, then think about the next step. Before you know it you will be half way along your journey and glad that you took that first step. Be intently focused on completion of the journey as well as enjoying the view (enjoying new health benefits) along the way. Learn to enjoy the tastes and flavours of real food which are much nicer than their sugared and processed alternatives, 'junk food'.

I learned much from my highly esteemed Taoist Arts Master, Professor Clifford Chee Soo (Grandmaster) of the International Taoist Arts Society. Most of his teachings I am *still* trying to digest, formulate, assimilate and use to build my own body of experience. With it, so far, I have helped many people to better health and it is quite strange to think that where I live, just a few years back, nobody understood the side-effects of changing their diet: e.g. Headaches and spots, etcetera, as the body clears the toxins and rebuilds. Now I hear strangers in the streets uttering the words that this book spread around ten to thirty years ago, "Oh yes, you'll get headaches, spots, (etc.) for a while, but that will pass." Usually they are amazed and grateful for one or two simple health related pieces of advice, whilst I am still amazed at just how much more the TAO has to offer (much, much more!).

One thing I am sure of is that after reading this little book you will need to think about it, so I have included the following advice from my Tiandidao student's manual:

"Wanting to consume knowledge too quickly will give the mind indigestion, so chew each word thoroughly!"

Chinese Names Pronunciation Guide

CHINESE - ROMANISED **PRONUNCIATION**
TAO / TAOIST   DOW / DOWIST   Dow (*ow* as in "*owl*")
CH'ANG MING   ZHANG MING   Chaah-ng Min
CH'I KUNG   QIGONG   Chee Gong
T'AI CHI CH'UAN   TAI JI QUAN   Tie Jee Chew-ann
T'IEN TI TAO*   TÍAN DÈ DÔW   Tee-an Dee Dow
KUOSHU   GÓSHU   Go-shoo
KUNG-FU   GŪNGFU   Gong-foo, Gung-fu or Kung-fu.

Basic Meanings

Tao = The Way / Nature's Way / Path / Natural Way.
Ch'ang Ming: Long Life.
Ch'i Kung: Energy Training.
T'ai Chi Ch'uan: Supreme Polarity (Tao) Boxing Exercises.
T'ien Ti Tao: The Way of Heaven & Earth.
Kung Fu: Person of trained Skills / Person Training hard to acquire skills.
Kuoshu: Chinese National [Traditional] Arts (Includes Calligraphy, Diet, Healing, Herbs and Art as well as Kung-fu & T'ai Chi Ch'uan. a.k.a. "The Five Excellences")
Wu-shu: (lit.) To Stop a Spear / Martial Arts.

There are many other names that may crop up both within this text and others, but the above is enough to get you familiar with the basics.

*T'ien Ti Tao (Tiandidao) or 'Way of Heaven & Earth' is the copyright name of the author's system of Traditional Chinese Taoist Arts and includes holistic aspects of the self-defence, self-development, healing and health Arts presented in a way which is better for westerners to understand but still preserving the respect for the traditions of China. T'ien Ti Tao has been thoroughly tested and accepted by the International Chinese Kuoshu Federation (I.C.K.F.) of China as "Genuine Traditional Chinese Arts".

TAO SCIENCE
The Supreme Ultimate

It is no coincidence that you are reading this book. You did not pick it up by accident or chance - it was your destiny to do so. As we get older we accept more and more of the many things which come into our lives and which we call 'fate'. Fate has been my accomplice all of my life. My destiny is clear to me and others who know me well - it always has been. Let me explain. To some the explanations may seem a little offbeat or unusual, others may say "Ah, I told you so!", but just accept it for we know what we know and feel what we feel. Just as surely as we know the difference between pain and pleasure we also know when something is happening in a particular way and what we should do.

As a very young child of 3, I used to have this feeling of not wanting to be here; 'here' as in on this planet. My Western Indian Spirit Guide told me I had to stay and had important work to do. As I grew older and long, long before the Martial Arts were heard of in the U.K., and before we had television or even books about martial arts, I used to 'shadow box', as my Uncle Bob called it. The name 'shadow boxing' is associated with English Boxing, but what I did was Chinese Boxing, T'ai Chi Ch'uan to be precise. How come I do not know, we can only assume or presume that it comes down to such things as past lives. On rainy days when it was not possible to play out I used to do 'strange' twisting, turning movements with my arms, legs and waist, which I knew to be fighting techniques. T'ai Chi Ch'uan uses such movements to deflect an attack and neutralise an attacker's force, then turns that force against the attacker by leading them off balance; something which later confounded many school bullies! When I was about 16, I was walking with a friend on Regent Road in Great Yarmouth, it was very busy as we had a warm Springtime holiday weekend. Through the crowds I became aware of a Gypsy woman, she seemed to be frantically looking for something or someone. She saw us and made a bee-line for us, apologising for stopping us and asking "Could I see your hand please?" My friend held out his hand and she looked. Then she asked me. I help out my left hand, which she held and examined, but then looked me in the eye and said "No, your right hand please." She then held and carefully examined my right hand. She looked at the edge by the little finger and told me how many children I would have – at 16 that was a bit bewildering – and then she looked carefully at the palm. "See? See the Star?" She pointed to where lines crossed on my palm to form a six-pointed star. I shrugged. "That is a sign. You are going to be involved in healing and great energy work." My pal looked at me in complete blankness, not understanding, but I just accepted what she said, even though I was still too young to understand. "Thank you so much." She said sincerely as she held and shook my hand. "I'm so sorry to have stopped you. It was a pleasure to meet you." and with that she left. She must have been what they call "a true Romany" woman. Later on I met Maddy, a friend of my sisters, her mother was "true Romany" with amazing seeing powers, and Maddy could read palms too, much to her regret, if she saw deaths or unfortunate events! My life has been filled with spiritual events, guides and serious accident preventions, so no matter what else I think I would rather be doing, I have learned to accept "my Way" and just get on with it.

As I grew older I was extremely aware of the conflicts of humankind and wondered why: Why so many wars? Why do men and women squabble so pointlessly? Why so much illness? Why do men and women do so many futile and worthless things in the name of progress? At school I was punished for asking too many questions, hit with the cane for pointing out the teacher's mistakes, stood up against unjust behaviour towards my fellow pupils or for correcting teacher's misinterpretations of things such as words in the dictionary. In my teens I was quite a 'rebel' and was even more determined to get to the bottom of the problems and find out why all of these problems besieged humankind. It became apparent that I had protection of some kind, call it what you like - some would call it a 'Guardian Angel' and in the ancient Eastern Arts we call them what they are, a 'Guide'. My Guide/s saved me many times from 'would be' fatal accidents or other calamities. Nevertheless, my life was far from smooth and troubled waters ran very deep most of the time. I could tell that all that happened was meant to be, it was clearly no good fighting it, as I had tried really hard to change directions on many occasions. It never worked. I knew from my early years that I had to write books, and that philosophy and lifestyle had to come into it. The more that happened the more became clear and my life unfurled like a long roll of material with clearly marked patterns upon it that some unseen tailor was cutting out, making a suit of future clothes for me.

The moral of this story is that life, on Earth, is never easy. There is no "free ride" and no easy time of it. We are here for a purpose and that purpose is to learn. However, obstacles are plenty and one of these is lifestyle. Our lifestyle can seemingly made more easy by eating ready prepared junk foods, the sort of stuff you see in fast-food shops in every town, every city, and every country. This temptation, plus sweets and the like, can be your downfall.

Here I shall pass on to you an old Japanese saying which derived from the Smithy who forged Japanese Samurai swords, renown for their lasting cutting ability, because I know that you have probably also had quite a hard life at times too: sadly a general condition of the human race:

> "A piece of steel has to be heated, beaten and folded many times before it can become a useful tool!"

My own studies became deeply involved with human psychology, philosophy and all things unexplained; although I could not see what all the fuss was about, for most things to me are as normal as breathing. As I studied I obviously developed theories. These theories needed to be verified by evidence of other people also thinking 'exactly' along the same lines. On far too many occasions to remember I used to be walking around Great Yarmouth, not long after having one of these theories. Suddenly my attentions would be 'grabbed' and I was invisibly steered towards a bookshop by some unseen guide: just as though someone was leading me across the road by pulling my ear or nose that way, and into a shop. I would be drawn to the book department and then the relevant section. One book would seem to stand out on the shelf, even though it was slotted in amongst the others. Picking it up it would open at a particular page and, without browsing, I would find myself looking at text in this new book which actually verified my theories. Satisfied, or at least amused, I would toddle off and carry on with my studies. This happened frequently with bookshops, libraries and even at other people's houses. It became very common, as did meeting the right people at the right time, for whatever purpose it was. Likewise it became just as common to be there for others; not all others, just those whose lives I could have the right effect upon. These things do not change. This is my "Tao", my Way or Path in life.

Having picked up this book, you are the same and this is part of our inter-relationship, our shared wealth and development. The Taoist Sages of long ago were less distracted than most people of today. They had peace, quiet and Nature surrounding them in the wondrous mountain regions of China. They were in a position far better suited to communicate with Nature, far less stressful and easier to become 'in tune', therefore enlightened as to the workings of Nature and the T'ai Chi, or 'Supreme Ultimate' as it is in translation and meaning Tao, The Way.

UNIVERSAL OBSERVATIONS

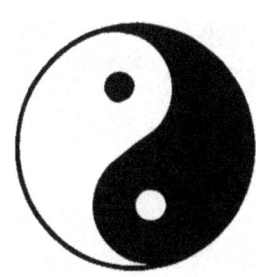

Taoist teaching methods are quite simple, even though they are still complex. By using images and descriptions, like Yang/Yin: Yang (positive, light, out-going and male principle), Yin (negative, dark, returning and female principle), simple images can be related to one and other about the Divine Works of the Universe and all within it, including our lives and all surrounding them. The energies of the Universe emanate from the centre and radiate outwards - they are Yang forces. There is more information about the Taoist Philosophy and its clever graphic symbols in the book 'Practical Philosophy of Tao – For schools and individuals' (same author).

According to the observations of the Taoists there are stages of development that we go through. There are stages that the Earth and the Human Culture go through, we are in a period of transformation at present. These stages progress for people in seven year phases for females and eight year phases for males. They are a rough guide only and cannot account for one hundred percent, for like the symbol of Yin and Yang (the image like a black droplet and a white droplet circling around each other) these are not all black or all white. There are some exceptions, especially those who follow the Taoist arts for health and longevity, for they may keep their hair longer and enjoy a firmer body, remain more active and keep healthy sexual relationships into later life. This is why this diet or regime is called Ch'ang Ming – meaning 'Long Life'. It is a way of staying healthier, living longer and enjoying life far more than you would if you made yourself ill.

We live in age of ridicule, people who study or practice one thing and who try to undermine those who do something different, even if the critic has no knowledge of what he/she is criticising. Social Media platforms (developed since after the first copy of this book) are a prime example of this behaviour. People calling someone "a Facebook expert!" (laughing emoji) without even knowing their target's background or studies. The ironically named "social" media is full of such insulting uneducated people.

With this born in mind, I would like you to understand that the table below is built from hundreds of years of observations, comparisons between physicians, people involved who were asked about their "condition" at various ages, and more. This is not some made-up, fantasy advertising theme such as you may be used to seeing these days to promote some newly invented business. This is factually based on hundreds of years of surveys, logging and note comparison. Scientific.

WOMEN (7 year stages):
At birth she is Yin.
At 7 the growth of her hair and teeth are prominent.
At 14 she starts to menstruate and is able to bear children.
At 21 she is fully developed physically and is at her prime.
At 28 her body is firm and she is thriving.
At 35 her face begins to wrinkle and her hair thins.
At 42 her hair begins to grey and her arteries start to harden.
At 49 her menstruation should cease and her child bearing potential gone.
At 56 her hair begins to whiten and she is less active.
At 63 she begins to turn Yang in her mental state.

MEN (8 year stages):
At birth he is Yang.
At 8 he loses his baby teeth.
At 16 his semen secretions are mature.
At 24 he is fully grown physically.
At 32 his muscles should be in peak condition.
At 40 his hair thins and his sexuality may weaken.
At 48 his skin begins to wrinkle and the teeth to weaken.
At 56 his testes slowly diminish and his hair begins to grey.
At 64 his mental state begins to turn Yin.

Whether or not any of us recognise or fit the patterns above, it serves to remind us that time rolls on relentlessly and we will face changes within ourselves: changes we could never have imagined when younger! We cannot afford to waste time on futile fun and frivolity *before* we get our problems sorted out.

First we should strive to cure our ills, whatever they may be, even unseen ones, and then being in a better state of body and mind, we can have fun later and appreciate it more. The older one gets the more most people will be set in their ways, thus making change more difficult to come to terms with. An old Chinese adage states about time and change, 'The only thing which remains constant is change'. Therefore the wise man or woman will deal with matters whilst youth is on their side. Time is the thief we cannot bar from our home.

Prophecies.
During training sessions in the late 1970's Professor Chee Soo quoted from one of his books, "Within 200 hundred years there are going to be great changes in this world of ours because time and energy are slowly moving into a flux of alteration". He went on to add that "China could become to be the number-one nation of the world", and that women would become leaders in many professions and politics. He also said that whatever the future may hold "we cannot stop the fulfilment of the Tao", so we must learn to accept the inevitable. This was said around 1978, and how right it seems so far.

[Edit: here we are in 2021 and "Wow! That was some prophecy!"]

Taoist Sages also laid down the guidelines for reincarnation and spiritual development. These are seven reincarnations for women and eight for men (see page above), women being assumed to be spiritually stronger than men because of their child bearing potential and maternal instincts. It is also *assumed* that most women will be more compassionate because of this and therefore have a head start: pending mental health, of course. The list below relates to the Seven Planes to Heaven, or the 'control centre' of the Universe as Lao Bah called it. We start off on the Earth plane of existence, or 'base'. Most of our incarnations are thought to be lived out on the planet Earth. As we begin there will be many distractions and temptations to get involved in personal activities, petty politics, and petty sexist issues and so on. The more highly evolved we become the less these things matter. Sometimes a soul can be reincarnated and be distracted by personal pleasure activities or other petty pursuits, or lose its way generally, an earthly teacher or guide is then needed to show the true path. As we get higher on the incarnate ladder such things as gender wars, world travel and material wealth become far less important. In Heaven there are no males/females, just beings. Men and women in this life, here and now, should expend their energies on learning to cooperate, not squabble over childish issues about personal, egotistic or superiority struggles. Like Yin and Yang, each does their part and men are just men, women are just women, it is nothing more than a convenience for physical reproduction.

The 'Seven Planes to Heaven'

Taoist Philosophical life levels are listed in reverse, as follows:
1) Heaven or Universal Centre.
2) The Celestial Orbit.
3) The Astral or Stellar Plane.
4) The Stratosphere.
5) The Magnetic Belt.
6) The Atmospheric Field.
7) The Earth.

The missing eighth level being accounted for by man's extra span on the Earth. The 'ladder' is said to represent our spiritual development during our incarnations here on the planet Earth. The often misunderstood concept about Taoists being alchemists who sought to transform base metal into gold is quite silly. Alchemy just means that you try to transform a 'base substance' into a higher state. In this instance we are talking about spiritual and bodily alchemy, so we are trying to improve the strength and quality of our body, mind and spirit. The only way we can do that is to begin work now, starting with diet, and not waste time. As stated earlier, time waits for no man, or woman. Many 'modern' people tend to waste their time on 'fun' pursuits rather than improving the things in their lives that really make a difference to the *lasting* quality, namely their spirit or inner self. True progress can only be made when we do things in the right way or order, so any personal development must take place in harmonics. The body must be transformed by correct diet and properly developed holistic exercise. In turn we can then develop the Qi/Ch'i, this will help us gather strength and good health. A better body will open up new channels in the brain and develop stronger links with the Spirit (that which has already seen other incarnations) and so we begin to harness our powers. Life takes on a new meaning and what were common problems, seemingly huge barriers, seem to diminish. With the changes comes a gradual giving up of unnatural things, those which are bad for us or cause problems. New and better energy levels come about. As the health improves in this way and we learn to live in harmony with Nature our Shen or Spiritual energy will gather in strength. This takes many years; it cannot be done on a short course. We cannot get it like a Degree or other common education standard, Tao has to be learned, practised, mastered and lived.

Where Do I start?

You start here. In fact you already have started, if you recall, you have already made some changes in your life towards the better, you bought this book. All you have to do now is to take yourself seriously and study the information provided. Study your diet, make one 'first step' by cutting out something which is not good for you and then reinforce that by including something which is better. Rejoice in your new found strength and will to improve things. The next step is to continue in the same way, one step at a time, cut out drugs and toxins. Eat healthier foods and balance out your diet the Ch'ang Ming (Long Life Diet) way.

The best way to 'follow through' is to take up some suitable forms of exercise which will open up the bioenergy channels (Ch'i Meridians) and these are only found in traditional T'ai Chi Ch'uan (Taiji) and Ch'i Kung (Qigong); simply because they have been developed in accordance with Tao. There are many forms of Chinese Boxing or Ch'uan-shu, sometimes called 'Kung-fu'; this means 'a person of trained skills/attainment'. Not all Kung-fu schools offer a system of training in accordance with Tao and any Oriental Martial Arts which rely on brute force alone are certainly no more than physical systems. A balanced system should use strength with subtlety, power with softness, slowness and speed, plus an explainable philosophical approach which is in line with Taoist theories and principles. Students of both sex and all ages will feel that they are learning something and improving their health and vitality levels (especially if they are also following the Ch'ang Ming (Long Life [diet]) way as well. There is much more to it than just fighting. Any fool can fight, and anyone can win or lose! As students of T'ien Ti Tao find out, the size of your frame or muscles does not determine the amount of power that can be applied, or energy levels raised. The principles learned help us to live our daily lives better by putting more quality in. As you know, if you put rubbish in you get rubbish out. Taoist alchemy is about transforming our lives and putting better quality in, hence the saying 'transform a base substance into gold'.

Many people think that the world is a bad place. It is not. The world is a planet made up of materials of the five elements. On the planet are animals, including humans. It is only humans that cause bad things to happen. We all contribute to the overall atmosphere and events on this planet, we are all responsible to each other *and* the world as a place. As you make those steps that bring you closer to the Tao and its natural principles you may think that the world around you is changing. People you meet may seem different and better. It is not the world changing, it is you, and as you change so you change the world.

Ch'ang Ming is the first step, the key to health, relaxation and better energy. Then comes T'ai Chi Ch'uan and Ch'i Kung and Traditional Kuoshu or Kung-fu. Combined with this are good thoughts and good deeds, but we do not go helping little old ladies across the road, not if they do not want to go! Good deeds are about helping others who are in need, not necessarily charities, which may be viewed by some as 'cash for conscience'. In the Traditional Chinese Arts (Kuoshu) it is not at all uncommon for Kung-fu and T'ai Chi Ch'uan teachers to teach Qigong for health and also practice TCM (Traditional Chinese Medicine). These Arts are all inter linked and it was felt by my Master (and many others) that one cannot be practised or taught without the others; this is because the practitioner's understanding of one is said not be 'full' without the knowledge of the others.

Many Taoists live to a very old age, in China some as old as nearly 200 years, but 150 has not been uncommon. In the industrialised parts of the world we have far too much pollution to reach such ages. With following the Taoist regimes it should still be possible to regain some of your youthfulness and enjoy the benefits of a healthier body, tighter skin and more youthful appearance, plus more vitality to an older age that you would not normally reach on a 'average' Western type diet with all of its sweets, chocolates, chemically produced, artificial foods and poor exercise. If you wish to live much longer then you must also move to a remote and healthier climate, if that is possible these days.

When I look around at all the self-inflicted suffering there is from poor diets and even poorer lifestyles it makes me even more determined to share this wonderful, ancient Taoist knowledge with you and everyone. The Taoist overview of the world is simple but complex, simple because all things stem from Nature and should follow Nature's course or examples. Complex because humans tend to lose the Way at a very early age, especially where educated to suit a particular country's or county's industrial placement needs only. This means that children lose out on their contact with Nature often and become 'conventionalised'. With mixed schools nowadays there may be some improvements as shared classes encourage some schools to teach more about different world religions and philosophy, This can have the effect of making children think more of the 'why?' and 'how?' questions of life.

TAO OF LOVE AND MARRIAGE

The general Taoist view of relationships is one of, 'if you are happy being together, then be together'. Couples are often brought together under 'odd' circumstances. Problems arise nowadays far too commonly in sexual wars, stupid arguments based on 'personal power' (ego) and other trivia. A man is a man and a woman is a woman, that is all there is to it. When we are drawn to a partner the worst thing that we could do is to start looking for things that could be changed to suit *us*. The perfect relationship does not rely on sharing all the same interests, jobs, hobbies or likes/dislikes, music or whatever, although sometimes it helps. The perfect relationship is one where you just feel very 'comfortable' with the other person no matter what differences their may be in personal lifestyle. Looks, height, build, age or colour should not come into it at all, so why does it so often? Because so many people are not balanced health-wise. Many more people are seemingly prepared to listen to the imbalanced prejudices of others rather than their own heart. A couple who are happy together and comfortable can quite easily talk all day, or embrace each other for hours, just happy in 'being', without outside interference. We should go with our hearts, not our ears, eyes or heads. The Taoist (natural) relationship is one of shared activity, not allotted according to some business-like list. Yin and Yang work in harmony and each will have something to give to the other as well as gain from the other. Is it hardly any surprise that in a culture where diet is poor and health is generally poor that relationships will also be poor?

Gender Mind Bender.
One thing which has become apparent in recent years is the female and male gender wars. Some people take it to extremes. For an example, one woman enquired via telephone about Taoist Yoga, also known as K'ai Men, she said "Why is it called *men*?" (with pithy intonations), the reply was simply, "Because that's what it is, K'ai Men, meaning *open doors*." She still didn't like the implication (in her mind only) that men, the human male, was involved even though the teacher was male! Gender is unimportant.

Sex and Age.
Sometimes a student may be surprised to learn that an older teacher of The Way may be sexually active, or as inclined as she/he was in their 20's. There is nothing odd about this or unnatural. Humans are not machines that switch off after thirty-something, and just because a student or teacher of The Way has a high plain of perception does

not mean that he or she is dead from the neck down. Far from it, diet and qigong, etc., keeps the body and mind healthy. In traditional Chinese Taoist influenced circles sexuality is a normal part of living: the human (or other animal) body is made to reproduce, so sex is very natural event and sexual attraction is the first part of any attraction between two people or other animals. Traditionally a Taoist man might have six wives, this was considered the ideal number. Why? Not so much all for for him, but for *them*. The theory goes something like: One wife gets bored, two argue, when there are three then two will pick on one, With four they form pairs and exclude the other pair, with five two pairs might exclude the other, but with six they are all good company and friends for each other; one may sleep or be with the husband whilst the others enjoy friendship and rest, they do not get bored, he does not get bored. It has nothing to do with just sex. Taoists understand many things, including the Way of Relationships.

Would I like six wives? That's another question. Right now, in UK, I will say "pass" as I'm too busy! Ha ha.

In the West sex is still viewed with a somewhat Victorian attitude and many 'double standards' exist. Some women see sexuality as a demeaning aspect to their development in society: in other words, detracting from their mental abilities. Other women appear to undermine this concern. Sexuality is part of life on earth. We all desire sex and the company or comfort of another person in our lives. In fact, sex enjoyed without preconceptions and emotional baggage is an energy (Qi) booster and can prolong life, rid stress and help the body to stay younger and therefore live longer. It is natural and should be treated as such. Women who are career minded should not fear sex or their male counterparts finding them attractive: nor should they use sexuality to gain favours or get their own way.

In the same way, male workers should not view female workers as a sexual object, but if the pair want to have sex outside of work then there is nothing wrong with that for sexual attraction is as natural as can be in this world and will always be a major part of it, for none of us would be here were it not for the power of attraction. This is not to give licence to indiscriminate sex, or sex just for its own sake, but a shared and appreciated union, be it fleeting or lasting. Taoist men do not treat women like so-called 'sex objects', nor do Taoist women treat their men that way, they just enjoy each other's company and what ever happens happens. Healthy minds and bodies do not pervert the Way of Nature. Simple.

Personal Enquiry
Think about the symbol for Yin/Yang, the two basic forces of the Universe; female/male, night/day, hollow/solid, pull/push, indirect/direct, moon/sun, cold/hot, soft/hard, winter/summer, etcetera. Then meditate on popular sayings, like 'my other half', referring to one's spouse or 'chalk and cheese', referring to the differences, or talking about someone's attitude, 'head in the clouds... or feet on the ground'. Why do we use these expressions?

THE SIX PART HEALTH TEST

There are a number of measures that indicate one's own personal level of health. Bearing in mind the old saying, 'you are what you eat', if you eat lots of fat you will be fat, if you eat foodstuff which lacks necessary fibre then you will be 'clogged' and if you eat 'balanced' then you will be balanced; this does *not* mean that if you eat 'refined' foods that you will automatically become a refined person!

A common short-sightedness among western medical practitioners has been to separate body problems from lifestyles. Compartmentalising the illness to just the small area it affects often excludes the actual cause of the illness. This may have been a poor dietary intake several months/years before the illness began to develop; this simple but fundamental concept is rather like thinking about a simple spot or pimple, these are eruptions on the surface of the epidermis which are in fact a 'release' of unwanted toxins or poisons from deeper within the system of the body. For something which most people can relate to we can use two common examples, one very quick in result and the other taking effect overnight: In the case of a person who overeats there are obvious symptoms which they have ignored, the feeling of becoming full up. The result is a most uncomfortable cramped feeling in the stomach and abdomen area which may later lead to flatulence and other dyspeptic symptoms. This is almost immediate, whereas when we eat or drink something which has 'gone off' or is now a breeding base for bacteria we get stomach upsets of a different variety. These are not instant but may take effect the next day or even later. By using these common examples it is plain to see that there are many ways in which the food we eat has an effect on the way we feel later. If we think about that on a much wider scale then the smaller or more subtle long term effects may come to mind; obesity caused by over consumption of fats and sugars; tooth rot caused by too many sweets and chocolates; artery and heart problems caused by excessive salt intake and/or smoking.

Our health, from a food and drink input basis, is vulnerable to all kinds of deviations. If you just stop to look at many of the foods that we buy from the shops then you can not fail to notice certain unnatural things about the contents; added sugar and salt in baked beans or spaghetti, carotene used as colouring, and so on. All of these additives are excessive and can have detrimental effects on our health, we already know that salt is harmful to the arteries, but carotene (the orange colour from carrots) can literally dye the body's flesh a yellowish colour! As to any other effects that excessive amounts of this substance may cause, we have no published laboratory results as yet that I know of.

All of the above examples are those of a more obvious nature, the symptoms of poor diet which are not so obvious can be more serious; they are harder to spot by the untrained eye - by this we mean anyone not trained in dietary medicine, especially Oriental which is far more developed than western equivalents. Symptoms may include sluggishness of the system and lack of energy, unclear thinking, lack of sexual libido, poor appetite, improper sleep and general lacklustre in work and play. All of these factors and more have been observed in the eastern hemisphere for hundreds or even thousands of years. As with the rest of the Life Arts, these observations have been honed into a fine guide for our benefits. Past Masters have not only observed the imbalances caused by eating the wrong things or under/over consumption of some other foodstuffs, they have also noted how we may correct the situation by counterbalancing the problem with the right food, drink, herbs or exercise and perhaps even Tui Na (massage and Acupressure). It is unwise to ignore that which has already been proven, but still many medical scientists in the western hemisphere have to develop electronic or mechanical means of testing time proven subjects so that they can get a 'print out' on paper which says, 'Affirmative. It works.' What these people with tunnel vision do not realise is that they want to see the results with their own eyes and cannot accept that this is what has already happened; many hundreds of people *have* already observed, with their own eyes, the results of improper or corrective diet for hundreds of years! If they stand on a pin do they need to wait until someone does a test with a piece of equipment before they know whether to say 'Ouch!'? Of course not, so why be so slow to accept the obvious, especially when it has been time proven?

Years ago people used to listen to common sense and experience. Years ago food and drinks were more natural. Nowadays many people ignore common sense and knowledge and also pump as much 'tampered with' food and drink and into their bodies as possible whilst also damaging themselves with dangerous sports, drugs, air pollutants (exhausts, personal and household sprays, smoke, etc.) and many more bad habits. It would seem that the more advanced the human race gets technically the more retarded it gets mentally. So what are these ancient methods of telling whether or not we are in good health or not? They all come under one heading, 'observation'. If we want to be more accurate and avoid any 'painting over the cracks' in our assessments then we should say *honest* observation. Many people, quite naturally, do not like to admit that their diet or lifestyle is bad, so tend to adjust their observations of themselves and make extra wide allowances for their little unhealthy indulgences. I like to drink beer, so I look at the protein content and say that it does me good. I do not have many (another excuse!), but even then, when the rest of my diet is far better than average, a little beer, especially a 'yeasty' brew, may cause the odd internal upset which may result in a headache (high blood acid levels) or mild stomach upset (too much yeast) the next morning. Fortunately, having smaller quantities and good ales, I don't get those after-effects. Even so, there are ways of countering these symptoms and after effects with other food or drink; fresh strawberries (Yang food) can counter acidity (caused by Yin food/drink), as can milk or certain bio-salts; Drinking two pints of water before going to bed will help flush the system and help prevent dehydration as well as diluting the effects of the alcohol. There are many other remedies for overindulgence or imbalances as well, including acupressure.

Before we go too far on that subject let us have an honest look at how our health rates on a scale of one to 18 by honestly checking the questions below.

In the pages below I have devised a simple check-list table process, based on an idea from old macrobiotics diagnostics, which allows you to rate each answer and put the score in the appropriate box. By adding the totals you will be able to get a rough idea of where your imbalance may lie. There are two tables, so both you and a partner can try it.

Use a soft pencil so that it can be erased, then others can try it too!

QUESTION 1 SCORE	QUESTION 2 SCORE	QUESTION 3 SCORE	QUESTION 4 SCORE	QUESTION 5 SCORE	QUESTION 6 SCORE
Use a soft pencil to mark this!				GRAND TOTAL	

QUESTION 1 SCORE	QUESTION 2 SCORE	QUESTION 3 SCORE	QUESTION 4 SCORE	QUESTION 5 SCORE	QUESTION 6 SCORE
Use a soft pencil to mark this!				GRAND TOTAL	

Photo-copy this page or make your own Chart: Get a pencil and sheet of paper, mark the left hand column (down), 1, 2, 3, 4, 5, 6. These represent the six questions about your everyday health. Mark your scores for each question to the right of the number. Do the same in the second column. At the end of the questions add up your score underneath, this is your personal score. Then read the 'appraisal' text below, which should give you a calculated evaluation of your diet and lifestyle. This simple test is based on the kind of questions and common diagnostics which anyone in the field of traditional medicine and holistic lifestyle would ask if being consulted. From this you should be able to tell whether you need to make any changes. Be honest. Most of us need to make changes, even those who are in better health than others. We all have to start somewhere and this is the first step of the journey, to evaluate our own lifestyle.

1) ENERGY: How is your energy?
Do you always feel tired and listless, fatigued easily? Is it too much effort to go out for a walk? Would you take up an exercise but can not muster the energy to get out of the armchair after work? Is sex just too tiring to enjoy? Are the demands of your friends/partner/family all too much to respond to?
(1 point for any of the above)

Do you feel tired and fatigued after work/sex/shopping, but not after a relaxing walk/Yoga/Taiji? Are you tired on some days but not others? Is the effort spent making love all right sometimes, but not too often as frequent sex makes you too tired?
(2 points)
Are you hardly ever tired and enjoy life, facing all problems and work, sex and sport with zest and equal enthusiasm?
(3 points)

2) ACTIONS: How clear are your thoughts and actions?
Do you get easily muddled or confused? Do you find it difficult to make decisions or react swiftly? Do you think that you have said something but are informed by someone else that you said nothing/ or the opposite of what you thought you said? If you drop something do you freeze with shock?
(Score 1 point for any of the above)
Do you sometimes react in reasonable time but are not always quick enough? Are your thoughts clear most of the time but you get regular periods of indecision ('it must be them, not me!') or problems you do not want to face? (Score 2 points)
Are your decisions quick? Do you react to physical or mental challenges immediately and can see what options are available?
(Score 3 points)

3) SLEEP: How well do you sleep?
Do you always have dreams? Do you go to bed at odd times but cannot always sleep? Do you get snatches of sleep for odd hours at odd times of the day? Is your sleep easily disturbed? If you go to bed feeling drowsy does it take more than half-an-hour to get to sleep or do you have to read a book to make yourself tired?
(Score 1 point for any of the above)
Is your sleep sometimes sound, sometimes shallow? Does a good night's sleep depend on how hard you have been working? Do you get to sleep unaided in between 10 minutes to half-an-hour?
(Score 2 points)
Do you get by on six to seven hours sleep? Do you fall asleep within a few minutes of your head laying on the pillow? Do you rarely dream or get disturbed sleep?
(Score 3 points)

4) APPETITE: How is your desire for simple and nutritional food?
Do you hate food and having to eat? Do you never enjoy your simple meals of wholemeal bread, brown rice or seasonal vegetables? Does sex feel like a chore rather than a pleasure? Is sweet food like chocolate more appetising than a good meal? Are you always plagued by period problems and/or constipation/diarrhoea?
(Score 1 point for combinations of the above)
Does your appetite vary from day to day? Do you get days or weeks when you just cannot be bothered to eat properly? Is sex a satisfying experience only depending on whether your partner is trying to please *you* or not? Do you enjoy wholesome food sometimes but like to binge on sweet or fatty foods regularly? Are you regularly, but not always troubled by period problems and/or constipation/diarrhoea?
(Score 2 points for any combinations of the above)
Do you have an appetite for wholesome food every day? Do you enjoy a plain granary/wholemeal bread even without spreads on it? Do you like to eat that which is in season? Is sex a pleasurable experience, no matter how much your partner tries to please you? Are your bowel movements regular, daily (stools medium/firm)? (Score 3 points)

5) REMEMBERING: How good is your memory... or can't you recall?
Is it almost impossible to remember people's names, birthdays, events and places where you have to be? Are things that are familiar to you difficult to recall? Do you nearly always forget important appointments unless you write them down?
(Score 1 for the above)
Is your memory fair, but not as good as it used to be? Do you occasionally forget things for no particular reason? Is it too difficult to remember odd appointments, although you remember regular ones? Do you only forget birthdays or special occasions sometimes?
(Score 2 points)
Do you never or hardly ever forget any event or appointments? Is your capacity to remember and recall past experiences good? Do you find that as you get older your capacity to remember gets better?
(Score 3 points)

6) ENJOYMENT & HUMOUR: How much simple fun do you enjoy?
Do you get easily angered at other road users or people who constantly do stupid things? (Remember that they are probably ill, too!) Do you get frustrated and upset because nothing seems to go right? Is it

annoying that some people say/do silly things and laugh, but you do not find it funny? Are jokes a waste of time? Do you find it difficult to deal with customers because they ask too many questions/make unrealistic demands on you? (Score 1 for the above)

Is it sometimes difficult to enjoy a joke; depending on what sort of a week you have had? Is it only difficult to cope with other people when someone has upset you? Can you see the funny side of some things sometimes, but not often?
(Score 2 points for the above)

Can you always forgive 'stupid' actions because they are 'only human'? Do you often see the funny side of things, even accidents? Can you laugh and enjoy good humour at virtually any time?
(Score 3 points for the above).

Add up all your points (You could use the box below). What is your score?

APPRAISAL

13 - to - 18 POINTS: You are already quite healthy. Congratulations. If you scored nearer 18, say 15 plus, then all you need to do is answer two questions more: Were you honest? If so, why do you not help others to gain a better lifestyle by passing on your knowledge and experience in some way? If you scored between 13 and 15, well do not give up, you are nearly there! Well done.

7 - to - 12 POINTS: You need to look more closely at the areas where you scored less. You are trying, so well done. Your diet is obviously lacking something. Read the rest of the book carefully for tips on better eating and feeling great. You should also consider other aspects of your health, like taking up Ch'i Kung (Qigong), Kung-fu or some other healthy recreational activity to charge up your system a bit. Exercise that has a wide range of movement also helps purge the system. Herbal teas can be of help in detoxifying the system and perking up your health, but do get expert advice and diagnostics first. Do not just try something because it sounds as though it *might* help or just because it is 'exciting', go for holistic exercise/s every time.

1 - to - 6 POINTS: You are in trouble my friend! Get help from a competent Doctor/Dietician and or Traditional Therapist, your choice, especially one who deals in the holistic approach (diet, herbs, exercise

and massage/acupressure or acupuncture, etcetera) in other words, uses the right treatment for the specific problem. Do not panic though most problems can be uncovered given the time and your willingness to succeed. Good health will bring you far more enjoyment than you have possibly imagined it could.

Using the right treatment for the problem is something which Western Orthodox medicine has yet to fully understand. Many readers were probably brought up in westernised countries, so were born in a hospital, checked by Orthodox Midwives, given drugs of one sort or another by the the time they were three years of age. Unless one of your parents or close relatives were into some sort of holistic diet and herb approach, acupuncture, or some other form of traditional medicine, then you may be totally confused by the concept.

Let me give you a really simple and common example of what is meant by choosing the right treatment for the specific problem:

(A) You have a headache. It lasts for some time so you visit your General Practitioner (local based Doctor). They recommend taking Paracetamol as this will deaden the pain and relive headache symptoms.

(B) You have a headache. You ask your local Holistic Health Practitioner what to do. They ask you questions, like "Are you doing lots of reading?" "When was the last time you changed your Eye Glasses or had an eye test?" "Are you straining your neck?" "Have you eaten X, Y, or Z, type foods much before you got the headache?" If you answer in an affirmative way to certain questions (diagnoses), then the Practitioner can get a more accurate idea of what is causing the headaches, so recommend the appropriate actions (without pain-killers.)

By completing the above questionnaire you will get a pretty good idea of what you need to do, if anything, to improve your health through your diet. It may be as well to answer the six questions again after a week/month or two has lapsed; theoretically you will have been a bit more aware of your general status by then and more able to give accurate answers; if you have any doubts in the first place.

There are many aspects to bringing about a change in your dietary lifestyle. For a start you have to be willing to make changes, then determined that you *will* make changes. Then there is the problem of change, trying to swap one unhealthy foodstuff for something better. With additives like salt this is not such a problem for there are many alternatives on the market which are quite nice, tastier and healthier; celery salt, garlic salt, sea salt, sesame salt, herb salt, Lo Salt and even 'no salt' salt!

Here's a little secret revealed: If meals are prepared properly, for the best health, then there will be a variety of vegetable with different tastes, then, with seasoning or spices, herbs or sauces, the "variety" becomes far more appealing than salt. (See: The Five Flavours)

Start saying "I can" instead of "I can't!"
Myke (Author)

Colour it....
White sugar (processed and refined sugar beet or cane) can easily be replaced by Demerara Raw Cane sugar, much tastier and better for you; you also need less of it. White bread (with bleached flour) should be replaced by bread with unbleached flour, better still with Wholemeal or Wholemeal Wheat & Rye bread. By taking a quick look at the ingredients you can compare one loaf with another and see which has the 'purest' ingredients and the least additives. If you can find a bread that is higher in Rye then it will be more beneficial in health, especially as many people suffer from wheat allergy or Irritable Bowel Syndrome after eating wheat flour products. Weaning family members, especially children, off artificial or highly sweetened foods can be a strain if they moan and groan at you. If you have to go out and buy their food for them do not worry, just tell them that (a) it's good for you, and will make you feel better, and give you more energy (they can help wash up!). (b) They can have what they like as long as they go out and get it, cook it and do not moan or expect sympathy when they are ill as a result! That should keep them quiet.

Tip: Kids are stubborn. Do not defy them white bread, for example, just place some small pieces (cubes) of delicious wholemeal bread on a separate plate in the middle of the table. Let them choose to put spread on it or not, and let them help themselves. Curiosity, at some point, will tempt them to try it. Say nothing! They will give you a look, enough to say "Well, are you going to patronise me?" Don't! They will soon learn that alternatives to the stodgy processed foods can be tasty, exciting, and may soon be ready to try even more alternatives. Once they do start trying and liking alternatives to the processed foods, when you go shopping, as them to find something healthy that both you and they might like. You can discuss ingredients then.

Learning about diet and health goes from a steep learning curve to a very gentle slope, even in later life. Whilst shopping with my youngest, now 21, I just learned that a specific Oat 'Milk' is a very tasty alternative to dairy milk in tea or coffee.

Too many illnesses that we see these days are brought on by poor diet, but this does not necessarily mean that the diet actually caused it in the first place. Chinese medicine shows us that are many interactions between the Body, our Mind and our Spirit (higher energy or soul). Certain illnesses may be caused by imbalanced emotions, as we grow up for example: child abuse, parent's problems (Divorce, rows, infidelity, etc.), unloved, unhappy home and so on. These situations can have an effect on our bodies via the bioenergy (Qi/Ki/Ch'i/Prana) and cause malfunctioning of the internal organs by means of the disharmony of the energy channels (Meridians). If these disruptions occur at certain stages of development the person concerned may grow up with a range of maladies from asthma to 'zits'; skin disorders and allergies, unstable relationship problems, dietary problems such as diabetes, hyperglycaemia or hypoglycaemia, immune system deficiencies and many more. Whilst Western medicine struggles to isolate the disease from the rest of the functions the Chinese Medical men and women have taken a more holistic approach. The combination of treatments can be applied to many of these ailments with startling results (startling to the patients but not the practitioners, that is!).

Consequentially this book is just one of a series which attempts to cover the range of therapeutic treatments more efficiently than one small book can. This way also gives the reader a better 'focus' on one subject before going on to other aspects of health and therapies. Just in the respect of Traditional Chinese Medicine (TCM) alone there are many avenues or aspects that can be explored and many ways of tackling just one of these aspects. In terms of 'therapy' the remedy should consist of the most appropriate treatment, not the most convenient or a single type, like acupuncture. Any good therapists or doctors should recommend an appropriate treatment, be it acupuncture, exercise or qigong, herbs, dietary, massage or Tui Na manipulation, etcetera, or a combination.

TCM is highly developed. Chinese medical scientists have looked long and hard at Western Orthodox Medicine and have rejected much of it in favour of TCM. This is not through reasons of patriotism but because it works, because it treats the whole person and because it also offers preventative medicine. I shall add here that before the western populace can hope to use TCM for treatment of their ills, there is something else that must be done. This is where this book comes in. If westerners do not change their lifestyle, diet and exercise habits, then all will be lost, or at least illusive. Nobody can expect to get better whilst popping pills, eating chemically induced rubbish, high fats, smoking, drinking excessively, being complacent or leading a lazy lifestyle. Does this sound hard? Not half as hard as having a doctor telling you that it is too late and you only have a year to live!

Addition.

This book was begun as a personal project around 1980. Since then I have become aware of some drastic changes within both our own culture and the Chinese Culture. Since the 'open door' policy was introduced in China and westerners were freer to come and go, and many Chinese have also left their homeland to settle here, a new view has been presented to me. A friend in Guangdong informs me that there are at least *sixteen* McDonald's fast food diners in Beijing! There are also many in other cities across China. Chinese people are trying to emulate the westerners and that, in my humble opinion, is a real tragedy: especially as they are mainly trying to emulate the American culture, which is in itself in its infancy still when it comes to lifestyle and social development; compared to China which has a cultural history of over five-thousand years! However, there are still many people with a sound and traditional approach to life who have also moved and settled elsewhere. Many of these people teach or practice TCM, Taijiquan, Traditional Arts, health practices and values. Thank heavens! Although I must add here, not all are into healthy eating or practice the healing or dietary principles, which, in ancient China, used to go hand-in-hand with learning T'ai Chi Ch'uan, etcetera.

Fact.

The human race needs to wake up. We desperately need to return to traditional values and healthier living. We need green issues not just to be raised but for plans to be implemented. Einstein once said, "If bees are allowed to die on this planet then humans would only have around four years to live", or words to that effect. We now see that pollution and global crossings by bee-killing creatures (in shipping containers, inter-continental lorries, etc.), are seriously threatening the bee populace of the world. Battery powered cars are not the real solution to this and are only being pushed because certain governments invaded Afghanistan. Why? Because there are tons of Lithium under the Afghanistan mountains! Big money. Economic restructuring of "green" Public Transport would be the greatest help.

Bees have been around for millions of years. Humans are killing them. Humans therefore are killing themselves, for if the bees are not around to pollinate plants (or give us wonderful healing honey) then we *will* reap the consequences and they will be far from pleasant.

Personal Enquiry.
In the west it is not unusual to hear of people as young as twenty years of age dying of heart attacks or being diagnosed with cancer, etcetera. Think about our lifestyles. Ask whether they are really doing anything useful for society, either locally or for the rest of the world. More important to you is whether the lifestyle *you* lead is doing any good for yourself.

Why is it that in parts of Asia, where people live in remote country locations and enjoy mainly fresh vegetarian diets, there is little disease: cancer is virtually unheard of and their response to the question of heart attacks is, "What are they?"

Why are governments influenced or affected by the thinking or monetary donations of businesses like drug manufacturers, chemical producers (Pharmaceuticals), Battery or Electronics, tobacco or artificial foodstuff manufacturers, highly pollutant industries and the like? These all contribute to a poorer quality of life in the name of science and progress. The answer to that one of course is Money, lots of money, backing and supporting the politicians in order to get their businesses advanced: this is called "Lobbying". Emphasis should be placed on those industries that improve health and the environment without artificial or harmful means.

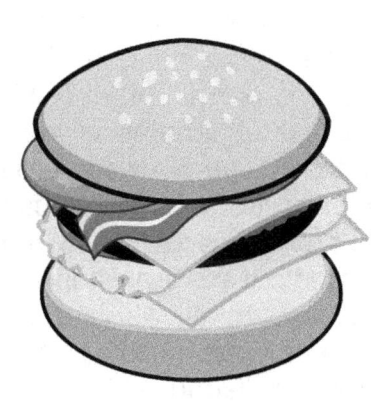

Yin, Yin, Yin, Yin and Yin!

THE YIN/YANG OF BODY LANGUAGE

There are indications on our body, head and limbs which may tell us much about the state of our health. For thousands of years the Traditional Chinese Medicine (TCM) health practitioners have, amongst other things, noted that certain shapes or colours are prevalent with certain physical conditions. Some doubters may say this is not likely, for how can the shape or colour of something indicate certain symptoms or illness? The fact is that we use this system all the time. We even have sayings that reflect it: 'Red sky at night, Shepherd's delight', thus telling us that if the sky is bright red as the sun goes down we will have good weather on the way tomorrow. The elements and our health problems are no different as they are all physical conditions with outward appearances. Take for example a summer's day: it is sunny, very warm and the sky is reasonably clear. As time progresses the warmth becomes 'sticky' and the air humid. The sky begins to cloud over, and then darken. We can feel a change in the energy of the atmosphere and we know, from experience, that a thunder storm is on the way. If we are sensible we take precautionary measures, otherwise we may get caught in the rain, or worse, struck by lightning, which may be fatal.

A common human physical indication of an oncoming lightning storm is that which accompanies heart attack symptoms. The sufferer always gets a small irritation in the left little finger. This is followed by a larger, itchy-and-tingling sensation which spreads from the tip of the little finger, along the outer edge to the wrist and forearm area of the little finger edge of the left forearm. Any TCM practitioner would automatically look for other symptoms of heart trouble; very red complexion, swollen abdomen, purplish coloured lips, red at the end of the nose, perhaps an enlarged or bulbous nose, a deep crack along the centre of the tongue and a smooth, shiny, red tongue. By spotting any combination of these indices the practitioner would know what else to look for and what questions to ask about diet and general lifestyle. A Western GP may give a completely different answer, depending on their skill level and what other diagnosis they use.

Whilst first writing this in the 1980's, I met an old acquaintance, one who has had many problems in life and whose lifestyle has been far from sensible in any respect. He told me that he had an '... itchy sort of tingling sensation', all down the left arm and little finger edge. His nose was bulbous, his pupils enlarged and his hands, arms and body trembled. He asked for an honest opinion, so I told him honestly that this appeared to be indications of heart troubles, as it was on the little finger Heart Meridian, and that he should take urgent action to avoid having a heart Attack: e.g. stop smoking, drinking lots of whiskey and change his diet. He told me that his doctor had said, "Don't worry, it's probably just a trapped nerve."!

My advice to him was to find a better doctor, one who also studied TCM (probably the more common Acupuncture) to get a decent course of treatment by a competent doctor (by using a GP with TCM training he would have access to the best of both worlds of medicine and equipment, something we 'smaller' practitioners do not have). He then asked my opinion as to what he should do about his condition. I told him first and foremost not to *panic* or worry himself into a heart attack, but to quietly contemplate a severe change of lifestyle and give up smoking, eating fatty or dairy foods and other problem foods. He thought for a few moments and then started making a hand-rolled cigarette; presumably to help him think about how smoking can cause heart disease! He ignored all the suggestions and a few months later was found dead in his kitchen from a Heart Attack.

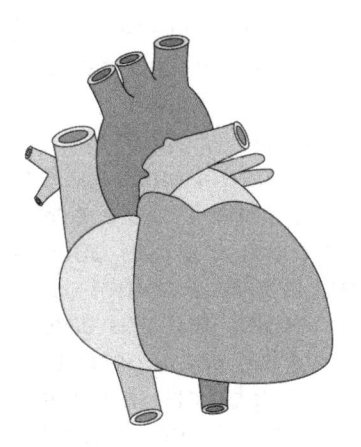

LET'S FACE IT

Other body shapes or colours can just as easily highlight factors that announce the presence of health problems. These tangible factors should not be overlooked by anyone in the health or healing profession. The problem with modern medicine (drugs and surgery) is that they tend to look too closely at the symptoms and by doing so can not see the whole; like putting your face too close to this dot ' . ', you cannot see the rest of the page. In TCM we look at the whole of the body and the whole of the person, body, mind and spirit; this includes their eating, drinking, hobbies, work and home environments as well as family or any other factors that may influence their health. All that you come into contact with can and will influence your health. A simple analogy is 'Bakers' Lung': a condition actually caused by breathing ion flour.

The face is the first part of a person we usually see. Facial shapes and colours can indicate a basic health tendency insomuch as they may be Yin or Yang, or otherwise balanced.

There are 'Eight Classifications' in TCM which enable the practitioner to recognise certain factors that might indicate illness, likelihood of illness or potential of illness, even long before anything physically appears.

Accompanying this is the 'Five Systems of Examination': touching, looking, listening, asking and smelling (body & breath odours).

This reflects the overall simplicity of the Chinese system. Many similar effects are grouped into a category and each can be defined further by other factors; sound, colour, smell, taste, desire, feelings, etcetera. By sharp contrast Western medicine has become too complicated and each illness or symptom is give a name, usually one that is a tongue twister! Ironically the illnesses that are categorised differently in the West may be connected to the same part of the body or its processes. These may be indicated long before the illness "shows itself" in terms of feeling ill or chronic. Yin and Yang reflect the two basic principles of the entire Universe and all within it. Constant study over hundreds and thousands of years has shown that Yin things are depicted by contraction, thin, cold, wet or damp, dark and decreasing. Yang is expansion, thickness, heat, dryness, light and increase.

Yang faces are very square or short. Thin lips are Yang. Yang shaped faces or bodies may indicate a tendency inherent through genes or growth to more Yang symptoms. Yin faces are longer, more pointed at the chin and rounded at the top, egg shaped. Yin features may indicate tendencies toward more Yin symptoms. It does not stop there, for every line can tell a story and those pimples or blemishes that some girls try to hide with liberal doses of creams and potions all indicate some imbalance or tendency within their body system.

Yin features may have colouring around the eyes, thick lips, long curly eyelashes and a long, thin nose. It is funny how the Yin features that are indications of bad health are sought after by actors and Hollywood film moguls as 'models of beauty'. Prof. Chee Soo used to say that we may as well look for beauty in murderers and rapists if we are to call Yin people attractive! Tall, thin bodies and swinging hips are also extreme Yin features, so what does this say of models who are sought after because of their extremely Yin features? Should we encourage young girls to be ill and unbalanced in their health? This stupidity is a hangover from the Victorian and earlier days when women used to strap themselves into a corset so tightly that their digestive system was cramped. High heels are akin to the Chinese foot binding practice. It is all nonsensical and women nowadays should have better sense. Too thin is the same as overweight, fatness and thinness are both extremes and undesirable. A good, wholesome diet combined with the right amounts of walking and other exercises will keep anyone in good shape. Forget crash diets and aerobics seven days a week; be sensible.

We may get many of our features from our parents, not just their genes but also from within our Mother's womb where the food she eats, the drink, drugs (including those from tobacco and alcohol, aspirins, tranquillisers, etc.) will all have an effect on our health and appearance both when we are born and when we grow up. Obviously the childhood diet is just as important here as well. Some problems may become apparent almost immediately whilst others may take many years to manifest, just like it takes time for parts to wear-out or go wrong on your car. You may be able to disguise thinly some wrinkles, blemishes or body signs with make-up and clothes but they are still there, they will still appear. Every time I see a woman wearing make-up or very loose clothing I wonder what she is trying to hide. There are, however, still tell-tale signs in the way people move and act, talk and react, no mater how much they try to disguise their appearance.

Please, people, realise that disguises do not work, getting fit and healthier does. There is nothing, speaking as a natural man, more attractive than a natural woman. I have seen women who are wearing no make-up, old clothes, and who have such a radiant glow about them simply because they eat well, exercise and also think good things. I know it works the other way, as some women who I have only just met, zoom in to me and give me a hug and a kiss, saying that I have "a lovely aura". That is wonderful: a sign that she is not slave to artificial things and is, as a woman should be, in tune with Tao (Nature).

If we eat artificial, we will be artificial. Use artificial make-up, clothing, and avoid doing what we need to do, naturally exercise (not Gyms or Treadmills), then we will develop.... wait for it.... Naturally.

The real crux of the matter is to recognise when we need to make changes - to let our body tell us that we are going wrong. If the diet is rubbish and the body is suffering, it is "telling you", so then change the diet. It is a simple as that. There are no excuses for a rushed and hurried lifestyle; you do not have to cram more into a day than you can handle: what is the point if it is making you ill?

HERE'S LOOKING AT YOU, KID!
A STRONG HEALTHY BODY is likely to reflect well-balanced health on the whole. If a person looks fit and their skin has a "golden glow" about it, their eyes are bright, their tongue a natural pink and without excess furring, then these are outward appearances of good health. Good health relies on more than physical appearances though. A cosmetic tan and a few weeks in a gymnasium may look good, but is no bringer of internal health. For this we need a correct diet, correct breathing and the right attitude too.

UNDER YOUR SKIN
Skin colouring plays an important part in TCM diagnostics. The skin is the largest organ in the body and as such a visible organ can tell us much about the health of the patient or subject.

MOIST SKIN may suggest a lung disharmony.
DRY SKIN suggests a blood deficiency.

PUFFY FACIAL SKIN (white in colour) may indicate Ch'i or Yang deficiency.
BAGGY SKIN UNDER EYES can suggest a kidney imbalance.
ITCHY SKIN suggests a condition called 'Liver Wind' in TCM.

WHITE SKIN: This can denote respiratory troubles (sinusitis, pollen allergies, asthma) or possibly anaemia. The blood is deficient. It may also be a sign of tuberculosis or leprosy. Glossy white skin that is almost transparent usually indicates lung problems. The skin may be "chilly" to the touch and the person may be adverse to climatic changes where it is cold or damp. You will see that most people who smoke have 'pale white' skin, or it may be turning that way, for it does not happen overnight. (Note: There are over 60 known chemicals in cigarettes which all cause cancer. These also burden 'passive smokers' as they are forced to inhale the same smoke.)

GREY SKIN: This is very Yin and usually denotes liver problems. It is common in the West, due to diet and lifestyle. The person who suffers may become angry very quickly, or they may suddenly change from one mood to another, perhaps becoming depressed suddenly, for no apparent reason, they may even cry spontaneously.

BLACK SKIN: This is actually any colouring beneath the skin of a dark brown and black coloration. It is nothing to do with a person's race, country of origin or suntan. Seeing these colours beneath the skin may indicate kidney problems (Yin) and an accumulation of unwanted substances (toxins etc.) in the blood stream. The dark brown spots that many call "beauty spots" are trapped toxins rising to the surface of the skin. In TCM it is thought that these spots are caused by over consumption of Yin drinks and foods; iced drinks, ice cream, synthesised foods, drugs and medications. Black "moles" are thought to be caused by the consumption of meat or meat products (beef burgers, hamburgers, etc.) and a person with moles may be apprehensive of nature. I have some small doubts about this one and think sugars can also be responsible.

BLUE SKIN: A blue or purple colouring under the skin is likely to denote too much toxin in the blood stream. The veins and arteries may look blue anyway, but not very much so. The consumption of Yin foods such as iced drinks, ice cream, tropical fruit (including canned drinks) and sugar will all contribute to this. Eliminate them from your diet. If the complexion is a darker purple, especially on the nose, then this may indicate too high a blood pressure. If the tongue is also purple then this would seem to indicate an enlarged liver and spleen and/or possible internal blood clotting: Urgent treatment should be sought.

GREEN SKIN: Green is seriously Yin as it usually denotes that cancer is present. If there is a greenish hue on the left side of the face it suggests cancer of the liver, on the right side cancer of the lungs.

RED SKIN: This may be confined to certain areas or the whole body. A red nose may indicate spleen/pancreas trouble, liver or heart trouble. Either alcohol or diet may be the cause. Gums are normally pink, "redness" may be an effect of expanded blood capillaries caused by drugs or medicines or even vitamin B3 deficiency.

Patches of dry, red and itchy skin may tell us that there is a liver problem or food allergy; cut out animal foods, all alcohol and seasoned or spicy foods in this case. Red patches on the face in cold weather indicate poor circulation, blood stagnation or perhaps an excess of blood. Blushing is normal and is not a symptom of anything other than embarrassment! Likewise the reddish glow on the skin of a newly born child is natural, as is a reddish complexion after very active, especially outdoor sports.

According to the Yellow Emperor's Classic of Internal Medicine (Nei Ching) there are five main areas that indicate necessary treatments:
1. A scarlet red complexion indicates heart troubles.
2. A red nose shows that the spleen is imbalanced.
3. Red on the right side of the jaw warns of lung disease.
4. Red on the left side of the jaw warns of liver problems.
5. Red on the chin signifies kidney troubles.

YELLOW SKIN, anything from pale yellow to orange under colouring, can indicate that there are problems with the spleen, pancreas and liver. The pancreas controls insulin and glucagons in the body, so any sugary sweets or drinks, refined foods (white flour, rice & sugar), tea, coffee and raw foods can all cause interference with this organ and ill health. This may be started in childhood but develop at adult stages. Yellow in the whites of the eyes denotes jaundice, an illness if the liver, the facial skin may also take on a yellowish hue. Excessive carotene may also cause orange or yellow skin hue.

According to the Taoist Ch'ang Ming diagnostics we can add a few more things to our observation list. You may already know these, as they are very common amongst people who live in major cities around the world, in Europe and the USA, due to poor lifestyle, junk food and unhealthy environments. Skin conditions can also be tell-tale signs of vitamin deficiency (see sections on Basic Food Properties, Vitamins & Minerals.

SYMPTOMS & ILLNESS

TEXTURE of SKIN: If the skin is **rough** then this is caused by over consumption of meats and deep-fried foods. **Dryness** is caused by over consumption of toxins, which eradicate natural oils. **Perspiration** is natural in small amounts. If you perspire greatly after exertion then you are over-consuming liquids and are overworking the kidneys. Someone who perspires just standing around or with little movement should seriously adjust his or her diet and liquid intake. If there has been no physical activity but you still perspire under the arms and the palms of your hands, then there is a problem with the lungs; although perspiration here is natural after Ch'i Kung (Qigong), static or moving, as you are using the lungs more and developing body heat in these areas (if in any doubt consult your instructor).

HAIR CONDITION
The colour, texture and general condition of the hair is not dependent on which shampoo you use or which hairdresser you go to. Hair is produced from excess proteins and nutrients that we consume, especially calcium, which is excreted through the nails and hair. Each hair condition tells us about our diet.

BALDNESS is a condition that is Yin and indicates an excessive amount of fluid intake (continuous thirst is a symptom of another imbalance). By reducing the fluids you should also reduce hair loss.

DANDRUFF is a result of too much meat and dairy produce. It can also be the result of too much protein, eating more than we need; another symptom of the opulent society, which consumes too much just because it is there.

FRIZZY HAIR & SPLIT ENDS are a sign of too much toxin. Again, the over consumption of fruits, sugars and synthetic drinks will contribute towards this problem. The same symptoms may also indicate weakness of the sexual organs or reproductive system, so anyone suffering from sexual "negativity' may do well to avoid such foods.

HAIR COLOUR is not from a bottle. The colour of our natural hair may be influenced by the diet. Grey hair or white hair prematurely is a symptom of eating too much animal fat, meat and dairy produce. The levels of fat in the circulatory system is said to affect your hair colouring this way.

ENERGY LEVELS naturally fluctuate, but they should be within a level and comparatively narrow margin throughout the day. If you are 'up' one minute and then feeling depleted the next, then up again there is something wrong. If you feel you need a sweet biscuit, coffee, alcohol or chocolate to get you going then you are definitely imbalanced. Emotional disorders can affect the diet, often setting in at an early age and being accepted by parents as kid's odd fancies or teenage choosiness. This problem should not be ignored. Long-term illness starts off with little things and gets bigger. Common dietary problems are often overlooked or ignored, foolishly accepted as 'my lot' in life. Nothing should be left to ride - get it diagnosed, treated and get the balance back.

There are many other things taken into consideration when making diagnosis on any individual. There are indications gained from lines upon the face, eye patterns and shapes, the twelve pulses, the sound of the voice, body smells (breath and skin odours) and energy levels. The contents of this chapter will enable you to get some idea of the complexity and depth of the Chinese system whilst being able to realise just how simple it is. You may also recognise certain symptoms in yourself, but before making hasty changes in your diet be sure that you are not jumping to conclusions. Always go and see a reputable TCM practitioner. 'Certificates' or belonging to any authoritative sounding organisation does not guarantee that he or she is competent. If you can, ask around your friends, work mates and family to see if any of them have heard of someone who has a good success rate. A good practitioner who does, say, Dietary/Acupressure/Massage Therapies may examine you and recommend someone who does Qigong Therapy. Likewise someone who specialises in the aspects of Acupuncture and Herbal Medicine may send you to the Dietary and Qigong practitioners.

The TCM Arts are very wide and holistic. A younger practitioner may have only experienced one aspect, or an older practitioner may have started late in life. The length of time that someone has been practising and learning the Arts is directly related to their skills. I started *seriously* practising the Chinese Arts in the 1960's and knew that there was more to them than just Quanshu (Chinese Boxing) and its associated fitness exercises. Since those heady days I have learned and discovered much about the human body, mind and spirit. After around forty years of continuous study and practice you may think that I now know it all. No way! Our beloved Taoist Arts Grand Master, Clifford Chee Soo, once told us in a Teacher's Training class, "The Chinese Taoist Arts are filled with thousands of years of study by thousands of dedicated people. It is epitomised by the old saying, 'The more you learn the more you realise how little you know!'

The holistic approach is very important when it comes to health because everything that we do or come into contact with effects our health and our lives; we are only now discovering the mass of facts about the many forms of pollution of the environment, both indoors and out, in the air and in the ground or materials. Likewise there is much to learn about the food that we eat. The remedy for the latter is quite simple though because the food that we eat changes very little. The only things which change are the way it is processed; production lines, additives, (sugar, salt, preservatives, flavourings, colouring), chemical cleaning or sterilisation agents used in food processing plants, wrapping and packaging (cling film, for example) and preparation factors.

Try to avoid as many of these "grey areas" as possible then our diet can only improve and our health benefit. Further more, if we try to eat more natural foods and avoid the processed or artificial foods, and avoid imbalanced diets which are not varied according to season or food type, then we will avoid many of the common illnesses which now plague or so-called 'modern' society. The answers are very simple - follow the Natural Way, which the Ch'ang Ming diet is built upon. With the backing of thousands of years of knowledge it would be difficult for a conscientious and dedicated follower to go wrong.

Use this section in conjunction with the others, study the whole book and think carefully about it before deciding to make any changes. With diagnostics it is important to remember that 'symptoms' apparent on one day may be only temporary. What we should look for are common occurrences and regular symptoms that are not easily mistaken. Therefore, just because you break out into a full body sweat one day does not mean that your kidneys have suddenly gone on the blink! It may be that you have just consumed too much liquid that day or two past. So think carefully and do not overreact. Especially important here is that you do not go around trying to tell everyone you meet that they have the symptoms of cancer, liver troubles or anything else. Leave it to those who are well trained in such matters and who can ask *all* the right questions of the patient. Even though certain conditions may be obvious, how they are dealt with is important. It would be far wiser and kinder, if you suspected a friend was ill, to ask them how their health is. Maybe even recommend this book for them to read, that way if they have any suspicions aroused about their health they can then go along and see an experienced practitioner for themselves.

> Grandmaster Chee Soo had this to say on illness and imbalance:
> "No one should *expect* to be ill occasionally... live and eat sensibly to avoid illness"

TCM - Traditional Chinese Medicine.

TCM is a worthwhile study for anyone interested in the health and healing arts. Too often people look at the surface and see physical appearance as the sign of health, but this is false. There are many more things that affect our insides, including our Spirit, than our outside. The outside reflects what is happening inside and a practitioner of TCM can quickly spot the difference between someone who 'works out' to look fit and another who is truly fit. Below is a small poem that helps you remember what each element in TCM relates to.

In TCM, Fire relates to the Pericardium, Heart and Emotions.
Metal relates to Skin (largest Organ of the body) and Lungs,
Wood the Liver & Gallbladder, Earth the Spleen and Stomach, Water the Kidneys and Bladder.

You will have more opportunity to discover their functions and relationships later in this book.

FIVE ELEMENTS OF HEALTH

Fire is the heart heat, emotions and soul.
All forms of life need energy to unfold.

Metal is cleaving, it's hard and it's cold.
Its uses are many, by Fire it's controlled.

Wood is the trees and all forms of growing;
Artistic, creative and spreading or sowing.

Earth is the soil and the mountains or clay.
The base of all life and recycled decay.

Water flows like knowledge, nourishing life.
Destructive, creative, pervasive and rife.
                                      M.S. 11/96

TCM & DIAGNOSTIC PRINCIPLES

There are 'Eight Classifications' in TCM which enable the practitioner to recognise certain factors that might indicate illness, likelihood of illness or potential of illness, even long before anything physically appears. These Eight Classifications are:

1. **YIN**
2. **YANG**
3. INTERNAL
4. EXTERNAL
5. COLD
6. HOT
7. DECREASED STATUS
8. INCREASED STATUS

Accompanying this is the 'Five Systems of Examination': touching, looking, listening, asking and smelling (body & breath odours). This reflects the overall simplicity and synchronicity with which the system has been carefully developed over thousands of years. Everything is related and everything can be traced by linking it to common events with which it is physiologically associated by nature.

The five systems of examination are:

LOOKING:
By looking we can determine certain Yin or Yang developments within the person. Yin symptoms may include being quiet, withdrawn and without Spirit. They may appear frail and weak. Their excretions and secretions may be thin and watery. They may like to curl up when they lie down to rest and their tongue may be coated with thin white moss. Looking can also include skin colours (see above).

Yang symptoms would be indicated by loud and dynamic actions, they might appear restless. Their face may be very red. When lying down to rest they may stretch out. The tongue may be dry and a scarlet colour; any moss covering may be yellow and quite thick.

As mentioned in the previous section, the hue of the skin indicates different health states. Hair, nails, skin texture and tone as well as posture all tell us something about a person's health.

ODOUR:
This is usually the smell of the breath. Obviously the smell changes with different foods, garlic as an obvious example. Generally the Yin

odour is an acrid (caustic or pungent) smell. Yang being putrid (rotten or decaying). You may notice that meat eaters have a very unpleasant breath odour, especially if you are a vegetarian and your sense of smell is more acute. Foot odour may also be worse in meat eaters and nylon socks will make the feet sweat more and exacerbate the problem.

LISTENING:
Yin sounds of the subject's voice are low, lacking in volume or strength. They may utter few words, their respiration being shallow and weak. Shortness of breath is common. Yang symptoms may show themselves in a course or rough voice. They may be very talkative. Their respiration may be deep and full, possibly even audible (normal respiration should be full, not strained, but quiet).

ASKING:
Obviously questions need to be asked to discover certain things as well as to find out more about the other observations we have made. For example; in Yin symptoms the person may feel cold and desires warmth. They may 'need' to touch or be cuddled by their loved ones much of the time. Their appetite may be weak and their urine clear in colour and frequent. Yang symptoms include higher temperatures, dry mouth and dislike of heat or hot places. They may be edgy about other people touching them. The urine would be dark, stools hard or constipation suffered.

TOUCHING:
There are twelve pulses, not one. These may be found on the wrists, both left and right. There are on each side three deep and three superficial pulses. On the left hand the three pulse locations are to be discovered just behind the thumb-heel along the radial artery. Location 1 is near to the wrist joint, two and three being evenly spaced back from there by approximately one finger's width apart each. The superficial three are the small intestine, gall bladder and bladder. By pressing slightly more firmly the heart, liver and kidney pulses may be felt.

On the right hand the three pulse locations are the same, mirrored. These are; large intestine, stomach and triple warmer and superficial. Deeper pressure reveals the lung, spleen and pericardium.

By feeling the quality of the pulses an experienced practitioner can partially discern the state of each related organ. The descriptions of the pulses are such as, 'wiry', 'slippery', full', 'empty', floating, etcetera. There are other areas that at an advanced stage come under the 'touching' header, there is the use of pressure on suspected 'Ah Shi!' points (meaning 'That's it!') when trying to see if a meridian's energy is imbalanced. 'Sensing' is the use of one's hand to detect subtle temperature zones around the body, also indications of Ah Shi points. An even higher form of sensing is one that is done from a distance, any distance! Example: during one of my Taiji & Qigong classes a woman who practises Swedish Therapeutic Massage asked about healing and Ch'i. I began to explain about Acupressure, meridians and Ch'i and the imbalances that occur. As I did this and talked about sensing in a broader sense I was consciously drawn to one of the male students who was standing around nine to ten metres away. As I explained that sensing could be done from a distance I walked up to him and said, "Like sensing this tender spot just here!", placing my finger on a point near his Solar Plexus. He was amazed, she was amazed and the others too. But it is a natural phenomenon.

This next section deals with the importance of natural phenomenon. Tao is Nature, humans are a product of nature. Humans, like all else on this planet, are controlled by forces unseen and many, as yet, unmeasured.

FORCES IGNORED
In western medicine, unless it is an obvious problem of the digestive system, the patient is rarely asked about his or her diet. Yet this is such an important part of the diagnostic processes. Having said that of course we must take into consideration that western medicine is still in its infancy stages, for all of its technological advances it still fails to appreciate the simple things, like diet; we are what we eat! Do you believe that statement?

Examine a simple parallel: Deadly Nightshade (Belladonna) is a herb, a natural plant. It contains a highly poisonous narcotic (potatoes, tomatoes and aubergines are all related to Belladonna and contain the alkaloid, Solanine) which, if swallowed may cause paralysis by affecting the central nervous system. It is potent enough to kill, hence the common name, '*Deadly* Nightshade'. Belladonna is of the same family as the potato; never eat any potatoes that are green, cut out any green parts before cooking! Another common plant is the foxglove (*Digitalis Purpurea*), this lovely garden plant, once wild in pastures on the Pacific coast, contains glycosides extracted from the second year's growth of leaves. These glycosides are used in Heart Drugs, one of which was called 'Purple Heart', another simply 'Digitalis'. Were you to brush against the leaves of this plant with your bare skin you may get rashes, headache or nausea. So, if we can accept that a small plant has properties that will cause such drastic effects by touching externally, or swallowing and digesting internally, then why should we separate these plants from all the others which are commonly consumed? There is no logical reason to do this.

Accept that all food has a 'content', some of which is good, some bad, some alright but only in small doses, some as an antagonist against the effects of others (as in medicinal usage of herbs) and some which should never be touched. Western medical practitioners would do well to remember the basics about sugar or salt and then expand from there. There are many foods which we eat, some may have a neutral effect; giving us protein and vitamins and/or roughage. Others may be high in certain elements, such as bananas, which are quite high in potassium. The odd banana every other day is not altogether bad. It is a 'Yin' fruit; tropical, not local to Great Britain (therefore not part of our natural diet either). It is this chemical balance we should be more aware of. Get it right and we feel good and enjoy better health. Get it wrong and we can suffer. The wise old Taoists have shown the way, now it is time to take heed.

CASE HISTORY 1: Professor Chee Soo once mentioned that bananas could cause miscarriage in pregnancy. This, like all things, I tried to keep in mind until it was found to be true or false, or at least have some form of evidence which could be substantiated.

A friend of my ex-wife's came to call one day. She was a couple of months pregnant and full of hopes. Her last few pregnancies had all sadly terminated in miscarriage. When she called she had a large shopping bag with her. On top were two huge bunches of bananas. She mentioned her miscarriages and expressed her hopes of a healthy baby. 'Are they for you?', I asked her. 'Yes.' she replied, 'Every time I get pregnant I have this yearning for them. I can eat that lot in one day!' She said. Then I asked some more questions and told her about what Master Chee Soo had said. She said that this time she would limit the bananas to just one or two per week and go for a wider range of foods, maybe even a lump of coal or two! She did limit the bananas. Her pregnancy went well and she gave birth to a healthy baby boy. In this case the roles of observation and questioning were most important.

CASE 2:
The power of some foods is so great that they should really be avoided. 'Rhubarb!', I hear you cry. "Exactly!", I reply. Rhubarb leaf and stem contains a substance called oxalic acid, a toxin. The toxin is more prevalent in the leaf but also spreads into the stem; that which is eaten. One particularly striking incident which was told us by Chee Soo was of one of his higher grade students. The man had taken drastic steps over a long period of time to eliminate all 'dodgy' foods from his diet. He followed the Chang Ming Diet with ease and with great results to his health and vitality after many years of study. One day he met a woman with whom a mutual attraction was felt. They got on well and went out a few times. The day came when she invited him to dinner. Rather apprehensively, for fear of her not understanding, he explained that he was on a strict vegetarian diet. She said it was not a problem and would cook him a special meal. The day came and he arrived at her place, flowers in hand. She had prepared him a tasty vegetarian appetiser and main course meal, one that was well balanced and contained nothing of a problematic nature. This he enjoyed. She then announced 'afters'. Through from the kitchen came she with two steaming bowls, 'I got this fresh, especially for you', she declared gleefully, placing in front of him a bowlful of rhubarb and custard. He so enjoyed her company and appreciated her efforts to please him that he said nothing, but ate the food. That night he was in hospital with severe stomach cramps which eventually led to a comatose condition! She obviously thought that she had killed him, but she had only poisoned him. It was a few days before he got better and was up and about again. Oh, yes. They did see each other again, this time she asked him specifically what she should avoid!

In this instance it was fortunate that before he lost consciousness he was able to say what he thought had caused the problem. Otherwise the doctors at the London hospital may have had to run extensive tests. Oxalic acid from rhubarb may not exactly be one of the likeliest things that they would be looking for. Even to a practitioner of TCM the aspect of questioning would be important, as the symptoms of poisoning are all very similar, especially when the person is unconscious! However, in both cases I feel that an astute medical practitioner of either ilk would ask questions of the family/friend that they came in with. Should this not be possible because they were admitted alone, then a bit of detective work would be necessary to trace their activities. Once traced, a picture of what they had been doing, drinking or eating, plus their 'normal' habits or lifestyle (in this case diet) might give the answers to the dilemma.

Diagnostics can be developed by studying the food of a familiar person. Try it for yourself, watch a member of your family, a work-mate or someone close who you see every day (but try not to breathe down their necks!). Do they eat lots of oranges, yoghurt, cream cakes, artificial drinks, salads, etcetera. These people are likely to have true Yin tendencies, beneath the exterior they may be jumpy, shy, withdrawn and easily hurt. Do they eat little fruit apart from apples, strawberries, raspberries and cherries, lots of meat (daily), hot and spicy foods, well-cooked toast, et cetera? These people may be aggressive, short-tempered, unwilling to listen or reason and possibly hyperactive. These are very Yang tendencies. Other factors may also play their part in our behaviour; our time and place of birth, where we live or work and in what conditions, etcetera.

Common Sense.
A more in depth look at 'elemental foods' will be given under the 'Simple Remedies' section dealing with Herbs and Foodstuffs. To close this chapter may I add a few words of wisdom? To diagnose accurately health problems may take years of training. It is not recommended that you attempt it yourself, nor is recommended that you become paranoid about your health. A sensible diet, avoiding problematic foods combined with regular exercise and fresh air should see you in fair condition. Regular meals, three small ones per day, but not too small, should be of differing foods to ensure balanced nutrition. If you feel that your diet is lacking in vitamins and essential minerals then adjust your diet before considering taking supplements. Supplements are also no replacement for real food, it will not do you as much good and your digestive system will suffer.

When looking for a health practitioner try to find one who is as experienced as possible in a holistic capacity. Otherwise you may need to find one who will do what s/he can and then recommend you to a known associate who will be able to compliment the work. Financial charge does not equate with quality of service. The only thing that matters will be their ability to give you an answer, at least after the first consultation. If they do not tell you what the problem is after the consultation and the first treatment session then it is a fair bet that they do not know; and if they do not know what it is then how can they treat it? There are far too many people today taking money for nothing.

CASE 3:
In the 1980's a young man came to me with M.E. He had been to several practitioners over the years, all of whom said they would make him better. One (to use his own expression) 'church based cult like group' claimed that he would be walking soon. This group has well known actors attracted to it from Hollywood and all over the world, apparently. After two months of treatment he still could not feel any improvement. They wanted him to pay more money for their so-called healing treatments, in total an estimated £6,000! M.E. is thought to be a stress related disease and therefore connected to the functions of the heart, lung and liver meridians. The effects are similar to MS and can be treated by selective diet and gentle but stimulating Qigong exercises, such as Pa T'uan Chin (Baduanjin), which is hundreds of years old and carefully formulated to open the meridians, increase the flow of blood and Qi, stimulate the muscles, nervous system and help fight off fatigue and infection. I had him change his diet, do the exercises and some specific exercises too. Within six or so months, he visited the NHS Doctor who had proclaimed "Oh it will get worse... you'll be in a wheelchair by 30!" carrying the hospital wheelchair under his arm. He told me, "You should have seen his face when I walked in all bright and bouncy. I did a high kick, put the wheelchair down near him and said, 'You know where you can stick this?!'", then smiled and walked out, leaving the Consultant stunned.

This kind of response is not too uncommon when TCM meets Orthodox Medicine! My Old Master had many clients that left hospital treatments after being told be them that they would not recover, but get worse, then finding under TCM they recovered.

Because of the very confusing and often overwhelming choice of medical and therapy practitioners around nowadays many people opt for their GP. Drugs are usually prescribed for the more dramatic symptoms, or referral to a surgical procedure. All of these options are low on the list of priorities in Traditional Chinese Medicine (TCM), for at the top of the list is what we might call 'preventative' actions; including correct diet, exercises and lifestyle. Next is proper diet. If followed this will prevent illness, but if one is already ill it will help strengthen the body. Next is exercise and Ch'i Kung (Qigong), followed by

Acupressure and massage, acupuncture and herbal remedies. Strong medicines (drugs) follow and at the bottom of the list as a last resort (for 'neglected' troubles) is surgery (this would also include radiation treatments and the like nowadays).

Why do Orthodox GP's *not* ask enough questions?

What this all should tell us is that we have to learn to look after ourselves, not wait until it is too late. It has come to a stage where we all know someone who has died prematurely from cancer, heart disease or other horribly crippling ailments. Yet more people smoke, drink alcohol in excess quantity, eat junk food with too much sugar, salt and fat and still foolishly ignore all the warnings until it is too late. When I think back to when I was a teenager in the late 1960's, there was a spate of drug taking, mainly cannabis smoking. Personally I saw quite a few young people die from various drug abuse symptoms, Cocaine being by far the worst, Opiates second perhaps. One thing that is different from the 1960's today though is the fact that '*we*' used to eat more fresh vegetables. I remember playing Frisbee in the park with a group of friends when we had nothing better to do, we all used to buy fresh carrots, peas, or other vegetables from the market and nibble these as 'snacks'. What a difference to the youngsters of today who mainly seem to consume large quantities of sugary, acidic cola drinks, sweets, chocolate, salted crisps and many other 'highly imbalanced' foods.

SUMMARY
We need to be more conscious of what goes on, what we eat and how we eat it. We also need to learn how to diagnose our own imbalances and check them before they worsen or become health, family, friend, or even life threatening!

As far as manufacture or retail of food goes they will never supply anything decent unless there is a demand for it. In the UK we have seen food stores like Iceland lead the way by selling no GM (Genetically Modified) corn/maize. However, they do sell other foods which are laden with 'E' number additives or fat loaded dairy cream cakes, etcetera. Other supermarket chains sell lots of produce which is manufactured, processed, laden with salt, additives and chemicals, packaged with gasses to preserve the shelf life, and so on. At least two of them are also trying to sell products that are healthier, at the same time as providing the consumer with "ready meals", like wholemeal spaghetti, or whole brown rice, with fresh vegetables and such like. Well done. Can we have much more of this please? Swings and roundabouts, as we say, you win some and you lose some. What we really need is for someone to start a store, nation and world-wide, that sells no GM, no fatty foods, no blue or red meats, no sickly (what an appropriate word) sugar and cream cakes and so on. How about calling it, 'Long Life Foods'?

Make your voice heard, write letters to manufacturers if you have time, tell them that you are one of a growing number of people who want better balanced foods with less additives and absolutely organic, chemical free.

You can find most food producers and suppliers on the Internet these days; which did not exist when I started this book! You can also find the UK's Department of Trade and Industry. These are good places to start.

COMPLIMENTARY EXERCISE

Exercise is called 'complimentary' because it does just that, compliment your health and diet. In other words, it looks good, feels good and does you "the power of good", as the appropriate saying goes.

One of the most important aspects of exercise is not the size of your muscles. Not the shape of your backside or chest, although most humans want to look "appealing" to their prospective partners, but the aspect of movement. The more of the body that moves, the better it will be for you overall. Physical movement on the outside will stimulate the organs on the inside; massage the internal body parts. This will aid digestion, as longs as you are not tightening up the abdomen to such a degree that you restrict food or waste movement.

Exercise also helps the body to get rid of waste, toxins and excess fats, as well as help keep the internal organs more fit. Yes, it is important to keep the insides fit, as they are the unseen machinery that really does all the work. Without them, you'd die. Muscles are useful to lift or move with, but they do not keep you fit, healthy or alive.

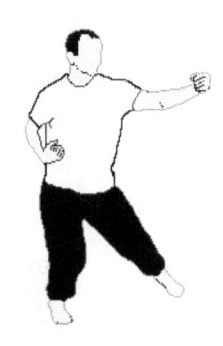

A posture from Baduanjin, the Eight Strands of Silk Brocade.
This fantastic set of exercises has so many beneficial effects and can be performed whilst seated or standing. It is ideal for
those who are convalescing from illness, for those who are fit, a lunch break stress reliever and body toner, a warm-up for Taijiquan and many other situations. These exercises are complimentary to a good diet and the two should work in harmony to produce far better results.

FOOD & EXERCISE

Martial Artists, fitness enthusiasts, manual workers and sporting people need energy, lots of it. This should be obtained from the food we eat. Food is anything that nourishes the body and 'Nutrition' is the science of food. There is more to nourishment than just eating virtually anything that is available - we have to achieve and maintain a healthy balance. This may vary according to our output, environment and, of course, the availability of good nourishment. The 'variant' factor can be stabilised by the intake of one of today's multi-vitamin and mineral supplements, such as an A - to - Z. The fact is that we need stable amounts of certain substances on a very regular basis. Age, weight, height, sex (a women's requirements are different) and energy expenditure rates, plus growth rate and level of sexual maturity are all factors which effect and determine the amount that we need.

When we talk about nutritional needs and daily-recommended allowances, we have to do so on an average basis. A detailed personal allowance may be obtained by studying the nutritional facts, the individual lifestyle, current habits and activities. Better still, arrange a visit to a Nutrition Analyst/Advisor or Dietetic Practitioner and let them work it out! If all else fails then you may find one at your local General Hospital.

Many Martial Artists tend not only to work hard but also become prone to frequent injuries, from bruises to broken bones' if sparring in competitions. Commonly it is a series of bruises, sprains and torn ligaments. Healing can sap your energy levels and may require extra doses of some of the essential vitamins and minerals. For example, it is now believed that boron will help retain calcium within the bones and joints, thus helping strength of the joints and resisting arthritis, etcetera. Replacement of minerals is crucial to 'top up' and remain in good health. When you feel 'down' and lack zest for life or training, cannot sleep well or cannot endure physical exertion even for small periods, then something is amiss. It is very likely that in any of these conditions, and more, that you are suffering from a dietary deficiency.

There are many bad habits around when it comes to food and just as many fallacies surrounding our daily fuel, such as, "a bit of what you fancy does you good." This bit of what you fancy may be influenced subliminally (e.g.; advertising), therefore not really what your body is craving for, just your prone mind. Local habits can drastically affect your diet. If you go to any sea-side holiday resort you will find lots of overweight, greasy-skinned people who are sluggish in movement and pallid in complexion. This is quite simply due to the over-consumption of that well known junk-food, 'Fish and Chips', especially those cooked in beef dripping or high-fat oils. Yet another common set of symptoms are observed amongst the people who inhabit other junk-food emporiums and eat copious quantities of beef or ham-burgers and wash it down with even larger quantities of sugary drinks (cola, etcetera). You can see the spots and pimples caused by excessive amounts of toxin, sugars and other dubious 'added ingredients'. In the past I have had first-hand experience working in a very large frozen foods processing factory, so have had far too close encounters with many additives as well as other factors, such as the quality of the meat and so-on. The UK permits the addition of '442' - ammonium phosphitides (not permitted in the USA) or **'E 127' enthrosine** and **'E 220'- sulphur dioxide**, widely used and **should be wholly avoided by hyperactive children and sufferers from asthma, kidney or liver disorders**!

Now, let me just give an example of the rationale on this. E 127 or Enthrosine. You can research the rest: The Internet has bulked-out since the first edition of this book, so you should find lots!

Here is a UK Guide.
Quote: "CI 45430 or E127 Enthrosine + other trade names.
Origin: Synthetic iodine-containing red dye.
Function & characteristics:
Red food colour. Very soluble in water.
Products:
Many products.
Daily intake:
Up to 0.1 mg/kg body weight.
Side effects:
Few side effects in the concentrations used in foods. Increased hyperactivity has been reported in a few cases, as well as a possible connection with mutagenicity (The ability of a chemical or physical agent to cause permanent changes in DNA.)! Enthrosine causes an increased photo-sensitivity in people to sunlight. In high concentrations enthrosine interferes with iodine metabolism. However, these concentrations cannot be reached through the consumption of normal foods.

Dietary restrictions:
None; E127 can be consumed by all religious groups, Vegans and vegetarians." (end of quote.)

NOTE: Although once made law in UK, have you noticed how E Numbers have been dropped from Ingredients on packets?

Did you notice that it said "Increased hyperactivity has been reported in a few cases, as well as a possible connection with mutagenicity… Enthrosine causes an increased photosensitivity in people with sensitivity to sunlight. In high concentrations enthrosine interferes with iodine metabolism." Did you take note of that?
Yet they use the term "Few side-effects", which, to most people who don't know might think, 'Oh, well that's OK then.' No, it is not OK, and far from it. If it causes any side-effects then avoid it. You have here a typical contradiction in EU & British health safety terms. On the one hand they are saying "Well, we know it causes health problems…" but on the other hand "… we will allow manufacturers to put it into foodstuffs anyway."!

That is what we are up against. Sloppy Government laws and even sloppier outlooks on health and human values. It is, in my observation, one of the likely causes of common health problems which the National health Service of UK, and others, cannot fix. They cannot recognise it, so how can they fix it? Diet is not even considered by the majority, let alone the content of that diet; e.g. additives. It could be that Enthrosine, and other chemical additives, are the main cause of Thyroid Problems, Immune System errors, et al. In Traditional Chinese Medicine (TCM), diet is one of the places to look.

YOU ARE WHAT YOU EAT.
To use an analogy, the human body and its fuel system is like the fuel and mechanics system of a car. If you were to put a tenth of the junk into your petrol tank that you put into your stomach, your car would not surprisingly develop bad starting, fouled plugs, clogged fuel lines and burnt-out piston rings and valves; not to mention some very nasty exhaust emissions! So, why do you insist on putting that junk down your throat? And why do you think more of your car than your body? It is not only illogical - you can buy a new car, but not a new body - but also it is detrimental to the environment and other people. By utilising a simple check-list of foods to avoid, foods to eat, essential vitamins

and minerals, we can avoid most commons ailments and attain a reasonable state of health and far better overall performance. The most difficult aspect for most people is the beginning. It is not just the will-power, but during the first few weeks of dietary change a 'system purging' process takes place. All the accumulated poisons, the toxins and other substances are ejected from the body. This gives rise to extra spots caused by toxins that are forced out via the skin, cold symptoms, wheezes, sneezes, diarrhoea and general debility for anything from a week to six months. In addition, if this happens to you, GOOD, I am so pleased for you; it just means that your body is sighing with relief as it rids the system of the toxic elements. After all, if you were cleaning out your car's system you would expect to flush out carbon deposits, caked-on oils, and metallic particles and even expect the odd back-fire. So accept it with ease that you are ridding your system of the crap and replacing it with new, cleaner elements.

Of all the animals on this planet, it seems that only the Human is capable of totally screwing-up its diet and eating all of the wrong things. Martial Artists, and other people involved in athletic endeavours, are one step ahead inasmuch as wanting to perform to their best. Not everyone is the same though as some are suffering from the effects of a poor diet more than others. With more awareness of foods and diets available nowadays, more people are becoming vegetarian and avoiding the chemicals, adrenalin and added tenderisers and hormones in meat. Many are also wisely avoiding artificial or processed foods, such as soft drinks and sweets, heavily salted or sugared tinned foods, etcetera.

As a Martial Artist, athlete or sporting person you have to be concerned not just about your fighting ability, for if your health is poor you will not be able to function properly, your muscles will be weak and your system struggling lethargically to support your efforts. It is at times like this when foolish people weaken their body even further by taking drugs to give them an artificial boost. The right diet and training will work wonders.

You may wonder why I keep referring to Martial Artists? This is because I have personally found that practising the genuine Martial Arts, the "Traditional" variety, not the Wei Con Yu schools or others set-up by people who could not be bothered to learn for many years under a proper Master of the Arts. The more holistic traditional Martial Arts are not only health changing, they transform the body, the mind and psyche too. My lifetime has been absorbed into the learning and development of the Traditional Taoist Arts. These began way back over 5,000 or more years ago and have been developing ever since: I am merely one in a very long line of Taoists who have kept these Arts alive and developed them: which is getting harder in the 21st Century "know it all, but know nothing, throw-away society".

The memory of 1971 stays fresh in my mind. This was the year that I discovered the Macrobiotic Regime when I purchased a small book called Zen Macrobiotics (by Georges Oshawa – Tandem Press). Beginning with the short-grain brown rice clean-out routine I flushed my system. The effect was probably one of the most powerful experiences of my life. My energy levels increased many times, my thoughts became clear, reactions faster and less jumpy or hasty and my appreciation of everyday life grew stronger. It was definitely better than any artificial 'trip' of any kind; no death-dealing drug seller can give you that one in a convenient capsule.

In view of all this, my advice would be simple. If you want to improve your life, training and overall outlook... go for it, start Ch'ang Ming (Long Life Diet) now: but only one step at a time!

You have nothing to lose; except toxins, fat, chemicals and other poisonous substances. You could just feel on top of the world.

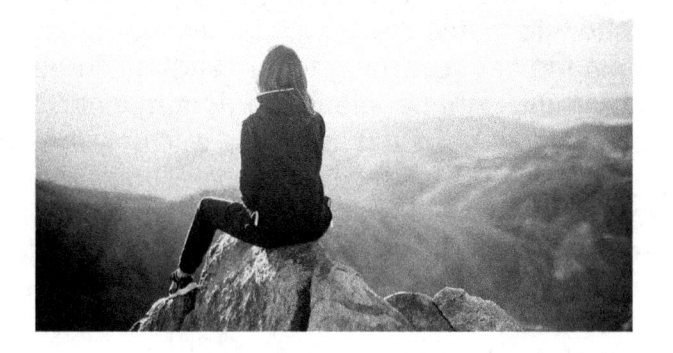

PREPARATION

'We eat to live, not live to eat.'

Many people enjoy eating as a satisfying experience. It can titillate the taste-buds and leave you feeling comfortable and secure, knowing that you will not be starved that day. For some eating can be a problem, a real health hazard. We are probably all familiar with associated food and reason disorders, like anorexia or obesity caused through frustration or boredom eating. How many are aware of the problems that may be caused through eating the wrong kinds of foods? For example, too many eggs will cause a build up of cholesterol, too much fatty food can create heart problems and too many sugary foods may lead to excessive weight, sugar diabetes and so-on. What most people are not aware of is the *balance* of foods. Each item may just look like a shape, texture and colour on your plate. Like most things in life, food is taken for granted as part of a hum-drum daily routine. In recent years, some connoisseurs have developed and spread their ideas on how to decorate your plate, making the meal look more attractive and taste richer or spicier. Television programmes seem to revolve around food, fast food and fancy presentation to titillate the taste buds, lots of fatty cream and meat. Little thought is given to the balance of minerals and vitamins that form such an essential part of our daily needs and determine the outcome of our health and strength.

The TAO provides us with all our needs, with a little help, patience and determination we can recognise all of those things that are good for us and then learn how to install them into our lives in a balanced way. Harmony is again the key. Learning to mix-and-match our food is as important as loving the right people in the right manner. It is good to be able to love everyone, but if you associate with only those who 'look tasty' then you are bound to get Love Indigestion! There must be harmony. If we eat that which disagrees with us then the internal system will try to reject it, if it is in frequent doses, illness will follow and we then need to recover, preferably by eating the right stuff.

Sexuality is part of the human form. Men are men and women are women. Problems will appear if a proper natural diet is not adhered to. We can see this in the Western Hemisphere as compared to the East of old. It is from the older, more deeply established Eastern cultures that we draw wisdom for today. Frigidity in women and listlessness in men are common among people today. Why? Because of food and drink and drugs.

Women are Yin, if they eat too much Yang food they become imbalanced. They may become more masculine and may detest the sexual desires of men and have no desire to love or be loved by men. Too Yin and they may be attracted to docile, feminine men, become homosexual or devote themselves to animals, especially pets. A man who consumes too much Yin food might become feminine, too placid and asexual. He may lose his will to be positive, to fight the good fight, be outgoing and active. In modern terms, he becomes a 'wimp' (derived from Whimpering?) and generally cowers from the problems of life. Whether or not you think that these statements are "against the grain" with today's ultra-liberal society is not my concern at all. These are simply the old observations of may people over many hundreds and thousands of years. The question that you should really be asking yourself perhaps is 'Oh, I wonder if today's sexually liberal, non-gender thing is anything to do with today's common diet?'

The old Taoist Physicians, health guides and others studying these important things that we call "lifestyle", observed many common things, some unusual things and some changes, all caused by diet and lifestyles. This enabled, if you like, a Catalogue of instances, diseases and effects, help and healing methods to be built up. Also a common data-base of what men and women were like, in a natural way.

A healthy woman is Yin: passive, soft and centrifugal. She can control her life in subtle ways. In terms of pathological extremes she may be too weak, negative, anti-social, escapist and exclusive.

A healthy man is Yang: Strong, active and centripetal. He should be able to control his life positively but without violence. In terms of pathological extremes he may become violent, destructive and cruel.

The remedy for good, natural health may be easily discovered and utilised. The difficulty lies in *keeping* to a healthy regime in a world full of junk-food pollution! First you have to discover your weaknesses, and then you can go to work on them. In the Art of Chinese Astrology each person may have a combination of five Yin or Yang stems. This can dramatically affect a person's outlook and is a case in hand where diet may be applied to swing the balance.

Example: A woman I knew. She is soft, gentle kind and intelligent. She has FOUR YIN and ONE YANG stem on her Birth Chart. Her reactions are leaning toward the pathological extremes of reclusion and escapism; constantly reading fantasy books, refusing to tackle personal problems and generally 'getting away from it' ('it' being problems). The simplest remedy would be to cut out Yin foods, such as, sugary drinks ('pop' or 'cola'), fruit juices and sweets, beers and dairy products. A small increase in Yang foods, like apples, spices, carrots, water-cress, onions, wheat germ, brown rice and parsley, would make lots of difference.

The Japanese have a word for this type of imbalance, it is '**Sanpaku**' and can be identified by those whose white of the eye can be seen clearly between the iris and lower eyelashes. Loss of primordial sexuality, aggression, unfounded fear, escapism and many other negative maladies which commonly affect our social sphere. I've sadly witnessed it all so many times. It is a fine line that we have to walk and occasionally we may veer from side to side. As long as we can recognise these wobbles we have a chance to rectify our state before we damage ourselves or someone else.

You can find out more about Japanese Macrobiotics and author Georges Ohsawa by typing in these words in the search bar of your web browser. His books have been a great inspiration to me since 1978 and I am sure that you will find them interesting too.

2021 Addendum: You can now find 'Sanpaku' on the Internet quite easily, with some descriptions of eyes, drawing or photographs, but please be aware the if you are looking at a person's face to determine Sanpaku, then that face should be level, not tilted, not looking down, or up, but straight ahead at you.

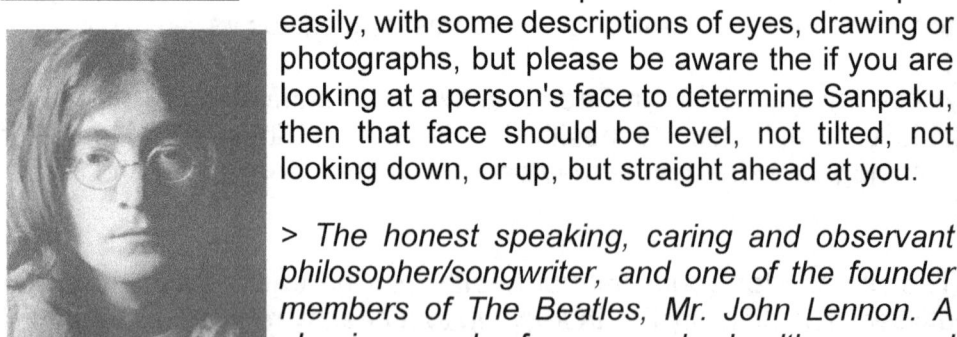

> *The honest speaking, caring and observant philosopher/songwriter, and one of the founder members of The Beatles, Mr. John Lennon. A classic example of non-sanpaku, healthy eyes and enlightened Soul.*

Yin and Yang Foods

There are some differences between macrobiotic regimes of one nation and another. What some regard as good or moderate, others regard as poor or bad. I can only assume that this may be for several reasons: 1) climate and changes in particular food structure or personal reaction to a food, 2) personal translations and understanding and 3) soil conditions. But this is no problem. In the West we have coined-a-phrase, "grey area", in relation to Industry, mainly. But if we think of the main types of food as being either Yin or Yang, then we can take those that appear to cross as grey. Thus, with a blending of White/Yang and Black/Yin we can either take it that it is well balanced or we can leave it.

The Macrobiotic regime is a method of eating and preparing food that may enable you to function properly, with the least amount of bodily interference from sickness, ill-effects of clogging and blockage, overload or deprivation. Being imbalanced will bring about a state of disorder whereby you will become confused and lacking in confidence. Get two people together who are imbalanced and trouble will follow. Balance is the key to a Macrobiotic way of life. Once you understand what is Yin and what is Yang, food can be ingested properly in proportions that are suitable for your own body. Macrobiotics is derived from Oriental cultures. The basis of Macrobiotics is the 'natural' theory. If you look at other creatures on this planet, or any other planet, you will see that they automatically *balance* their daily diet. Those with 'pets' that are fed on unnatural things will notice 'strange tendencies' in the animal's nature. For instance, a person (who may be vegetarian) will often buy tins of dog/cat food at the supermarket for her/his pet. How many times have you seen a cat or dog leap on a cow, bite it to death and rip out its liver, then cook it? When did you last see a dog killing a pig for its supper, or plucking a chicken and then cooking it? The meat that is in the tins is usually *extremely* unnatural for that animal: in fact it is unnatural to keep animals as pets.

The Japanese word for Tao is Do (Way), meaning the same thing having been ported across from the Chinese culture. Sometimes they describe its functions as The Unique Principle, which all amounts to the same thing, Nature's Way and the Power of The Universe. The man who was probably responsible for introducing the West to Macrobiotics was one, George Ohsawa with his book, Zen Macrobiotics (Tandem Press) in the late 1970's. When he was asked about eating meat he replied, "Eat only those things which do not protest or run away!" There is an old theory that by eating some animals, certain aggressive characteristics were transferred to the person. We now know with the aid of medical science that when a cow is slaughtered, adrenalin is soaked into the meat, along with substances that were unheard of in old China and Japan, artificial growth inducers for one. Adrenalin and other substances in excess can cause aggression and illness. Beef, lamb and pig (pork, bacon) are extremely Yin by nature, too Yin to be balanced properly. The 'added effects' of hormone injections, growth inducers, various drugs, may also cause untold damage to the human body.

General advice:
- Eat only that which is natural (No processed food/drink).
- Do not eat meat - it is full of toxins, hormones, chemicals, etcetera.
- If you really must eat meat, make it white and organic.
- Reduce salt intake. Use a sea-salt or a substitute 'mix'.
- Pick young, fresh vegetables and fruit for more goodness.
- Balance potassium (YIN) and sodium (YANG).
- Balance foods (Yang & Yin - one part Yang to five parts Yin).
- Do not over-fill your stomach. Eat small but regular meals.
- Avoid large late night meals if possible; after 7 p.m.
- Try to eat fruit and vegetables locally grown and in season.
- Blend your own juices, herbal recipes and cook them with love.
- Try to avoid allotment foods that are near main roads as these may be contaminated by diesel and petrol exhaust deposits.

The Orientals and especially the Taoists must surely be accredited with many wonderful insights into healthy living and prolongation of life. For instance, they recommended, many years before Jesus Christ was born, that it was healthy to practice exercises like T'ai Chi Ch'uan (Supreme Polarity/Ultimate Boxing) and Ch'i Kung (Life Force Energy Training) atop mountains, by waterfalls, streams or by the ocean and beneath lush trees. Only now are the slow, and somewhat detached from Nature, Western sciences realising the wisdom in this. Technology at last has proven that these are the places where the health giving negative ions are to be found in abundance. Taoist philosophers also stated, 'To gain the positive seek the negative', also echoed by Lao Tzu's Tao Te Ching (Daodejing).

In almost every aspect of living, from eating, posture to sexual practices, the Taoists were and always will be years ahead. For the average hard-working person though, philosophy holds no weight. They have no time to study its depths or fathom its reflections. What is needed is a clear and simple guide that will help them overcome the obstacles and put theory into practice. The parallel of T'ai Chi and diet is not used lightly here. T'ai Chi Ch'uan is not only a beautiful exercise and graceful, but also well balanced. It springs from the Tao and reflects the two polarities, Yin and Yang, these are soft and hard, cold and hot, female and male, light and heavy, subtle and direct, calm and vigorous respectively. There is a less complex T'ai Chi of foods, too. A harmonic balance may be reached by understanding the essence-nature of each produce. Quite simply some foods are Yin whilst others are more Yang. The correct 'mixture' of these should be approximately 5 parts Yin to 1 part Yang, this providing the right balance.

YIN FOODS: Liquids, milk, cheese, oranges (and most fruits), corn, wheat, sugar, pulses, potatoes, etcetera. These are often potent through the sheer quantity consumed every day.

YANG FOODS: Salt, strawberries, apples, spices, peppers, animal meat, ginseng, brown rice, curry powder, etcetera. These are perhaps consumed less often but should form one fifth of the daily meals.

The basic rules are simple enough to write or remember. What one needs to concentrate on is having the will to follow them.

FIVE RULES FOR HEALTHIER EATING:
1. Eat only when hungry, not habitually.
2. Eat only natural food and drinks.
3. Chew every mouthful really well.
4. Never over-eat or overload the system.
5. Keep liquids down to a healthy minimum.

If you have a problem that causes you to overindulge then a visit to a highly recommended health practitioner or a telephone call to a 'Care-Line' may be all that is needed to help you back on the right track. Reading this book will certainly provide you with enough knowledge, or at least some food for thought! Some people require personal assistance, someone to help them along. Whichever side of the fence you are on, try to let common sense prevail.

So how did our early Eastern cousins discover the properties of different foods? It is a fact that they had nothing of the resources that we have available today. They were not able to dissolve a piece of food in chemicals and study the results under a microscope. Yet they were able to determine the effects of each type of food on the human body and analyse its values. Mostly this was done by visual, oral and audio technique; looking, asking and listening. This technique seems to be very rare nowadays and probably accounts for the number of reported GP's who sit there looking at you quite blankly while you explain your maladies and still prescribe that you 'lay down and take two aspirins'.

The old women and men of the villages knew much of health and healing for they observed and scrutinised life. Though some of it was superstition and quackery most of it was based upon years of accumulative studies and 'putting two-and-two together'. How come most of it appears to be lost or ignored by most people? The answer to that one is quite simple. Over the last few centuries there has been a population boom. With it came a new technology boom. Every new change has helped create a society that has become geared to 'moving on' and trying something new. The 'old' ways almost became a swearword. Now we find that we have left something of great value behind. Within the modern medical profession we find those who are dedicated to 'its wonders', only a few are now wisely looking to the old eastern cultures for better answers. We also find some people being abandoned by the 'specialists' when they become 'incurably ill'! - Ironically some specialist doctors used to recommend their client to Master Chee Soo when they had to admit defeat, one recorded as saying "Go see the little Chinese gentleman down the road"! (According to an article in the [Luton & Dunstable] Evening Post 07/10/71).

Many of his clients were in fact recommended by GP's or Specialists, whop realised the constraints and lacking of the NHS's Western Orthodox System, or its dependency on drugs.

One such person was Mrs. Slow who claimed, 'I have had Multiple Sclerosis for 23 years. Four years ago I was so bad I could hardly put one leg in front of the other and after the last attack my hands were severely afflicted.' She continues, 'Then I came to Cliff [Prof. Chee Soo], I lost two stones, which I'm delighted about, and for the first time I can go out to work.... I'm tired but feel well - I've so much more energy, I can run upstairs. The Multiple Sclerosis Association in Northampton calls me the wonder girl!'. I remember that at a Choi Kung (Teacher

Training) session Chee Soo told us of healing techniques for MS, these included the wonderful Pa Tuan Chin Qi Gong set of exercises and Ch'ang Ming diet.

In <u>T'ai Chi Ch'uan</u> (often written for convenience as 'Tai Chi' or 'Tai Chi Chuan' – but meaning something completely different!) one is supposed to learn every aspect of health and protection in order to become 'complete' or whole person. The Chinese call this 'Kuoshu', meaning National Arts but relating to the practice and elevation of (1) exercise through self-defence, (2) nei kung skills like T'ai Chi Ch'uan, (3) Calligraphy (writing), (4) Art, and (5) learning about health through diet and herbs combined perhaps with healing skills: rarely some people translate as only three skills, but traditionally it was five skills or 'life sciences'.

Professor Clifford Chee Soo, gave us basic dietary guidelines which are said to be of ancient Taoist origin which go right back as far as The Yellow Emperor or before. One of the things which never ceases to amaze me is that in cases such as this, where a great Teacher of The Way is involved, most students miss the point, it seems. Instead of taking the dietary aspect as being the 'foundation builder' for the human frame, most seem to concentrate on the Taijiquan or 'Gongfu' aspects. Whatever the reasons are for missing this and concentrating on the *physical* Art Form they are missing the point – in this case the old Chinese teaching story fits perfectly - The teacher pointed towards the heavens, "Look at the moon", he said. The student looked up at the teacher's finger pointing. "No!" said the teacher, slapping the student lightly on the back of the head, "Don't look at the finger, otherwise you will miss all the heavenly beauty!"

The ancient Taoist guidelines I have updated where possible so that it may become clearer as to what food is and what it does to you or for you. It is not to be taken as a recipe but as a check-list of what is or is not good for you in general. At first the list may seem formidable, but if you take my simple advice of 'list and lose', just one item at one time, then it is very simple and an interesting learning curve with plenty of time to study and digest.... both the food and the knowledge.

TAOIST DIETARY GUIDELINES

THE FOLLOWING FOODS MAY BE EATEN:
01. All natural, organic and unrefined, whole grain foods.
02. Edible Seaweed.
03. Locally grown vegetables that are in season, especially root vegetables
    (But not those in 10 of Foods Not To Be Eaten).
04. Soya and Mung Bean Shoots (Bean sprouts).
05. Locally grown nuts, but not salted.
06. Only locally grown fresh fruit that is in season.
07. Low fat, natural yoghurt in moderation.
08. Small amounts of honey (local).
09. Cottage or vegetarian cheeses, in moderation.
10. Herb or China teas.
11. Pure vegetable oil margarine (sunflower or *de-fatted* soya[1]).
12. Eggs scrambled or omelette. Better still, yolk only (two per week max).
13. Natural sea salt, sesame salt, herb salt or soya sauce.
14. All dried fruit such as cherries, raisins, currants, figs.
15. Grain or rice milk, or if necessary, skimmed cow's milk.
16. Home made fresh fruit drinks [see number 6].
17. Wild vegetables and herbs (choose very carefully and only if expert!)

DO NOT EAT THESE FOODS:
01. Refined, processed, coloured or flavoured foods.
02. Processed grain foods; white bread, flour, rice, (also in cakes, etc, at least regularly).
03. Deep fried foods or foods fried in fat.
04. Spices, rock salt (table salt), excessive curry, mustard, vinegar, pickles, chilies.
05. Coffee, *alcohol, tobacco, chocolate and other sweets'
06. Red meats; pork, beef, mutton, lamb, veal.
07. Blue Meats; shark, mackerel, tuna, swordfish or whale   (salmon also).
08. Ice cream, artificial jellies or synthetic fruit-juices.
09. Sugar, especially Beet Sugar (white: processed).
10. Potatoes, tomatoes, aubergines[2]
11. Concentrated meat extracts or gravies/soups with same.

---

[1]   Soya is naturally high in fatty acids that could induce heart conditions. Always look for 'de-fatted' soya products and eat only in moderation.

[2]   All related to Belladonna and containing the alkaloid, Solanine poison), or rhubarb and spinach (both contain soluble oxalic acid.

12. Cheese, milk, butter, boiled or fried eggs.
13. Lard, dripping or any animal fats.
14. Any creature that has 'fat tissue'.

It is better not to eat any meats whatsoever; no meat is necessary for the human body to survive. The saying about needing meat for strength is an old marketing ploy: similar to that used by spinach growers in the USA when they came up with the 'Popeye' character; in the UK we had Desperate Dan eating 'Cow Pies' – I wonder if he died of gut cancer? If you want to argue about strength and vegetarianism then argue with one of televisions 'Gladiator' champions and successful 'Veggie' contestants, Einstein, The Dalai Lama or better still a powerful gorilla or elephant! Not only that it has been medically stated that animal meats and fats are very difficult for the human digestive system to break-down, they cause excess acidity, toxins and have very bad repercussions on the nervous and circulatory systems. The problem of ignorance of the facts still exists, even within the medical profession. I must confess, I even know of so-called 'Natural Healers' and 'Alternative Practitioners' who still consume meats, processed (junk) foods and smoke cigarettes as though they were going to die without them. These people obviously have not taken their studies seriously enough. How paradoxically funny humans can get. It is unwise to ignore health warnings just for the sake of titillating your taste buds, for if you become seriously ill a hospital diet may be much harder to bear!

A good healthy diet will not only cure most illnesses but should, more importantly preclude future sickness. If accompanied by correct breathing technique (Qi Gong) and regular exercise, like callisthenics, then one can triple the effects. More hopefully one will never fall prey to things like cancers of the gut. It is bad enough that in this day and age we have huge numbers of chemicals and fumes pervading our breathing air from factory outlets, farm sprays, diesel and petrol exhausts and even household sprays and chemical room perfume atomisers (read the warnings on the cans!) and equipment. Most of us with any sense naturally hold our breath if we see a cloud of motor exhaust fumes drifting towards us, so why do the same people insist on smoking cigarettes/cigars/pipes or eating foods that are known to be bad for us? It just does not make sense.

What This Book Is All About!

Ch'ang Ming (Long Life) Diet. There follows a table of foods that are either Yin or Yang by definition. This definition is obtained by understanding the contents of each food item and the effects of it; a banana contains high levels of phosphorus, vitamin A and calcium, but because it also contains high levels of *potassium*, therefore it is very Yin. Potassium is found in most foods, so deficiency would be rare. It works in conjunction with sodium to regulate levels of acidity and alkalinity within the body. It also helps maintain the correct water balance.

As stated elsewhere, this is not a 'fad' diet. It is not a quick fix either, but you may notice some rather drastic changes almost immediately if you change certain food habits, all for the good. We eat to live. From the time we are in our mother's womb we eat, or are fed, whatever she consumes. This is our foundation in life and can create a 'map' of our future health route: e.g. Medical scientists already know that alcohol and drugs can badly affect a baby in the womb, we know that the wrong foodstuffs or a poor diet can do the same.

The human body is made from water and a mixture of vitamins and minerals that are consumed, along with copious quantities of oxygen, and then processed and turned into various resources within the body (see Vitamins and Minerals). The body's own processing power depends upon the health of the system, which is governed by input (quality of 'fuels'). The body needs to have the right balance of foodstuffs, as well as good quality water and air. Should this balance be swung too far one way or the other then the 'health balance' is disrupted and pathogens (disease forming situations) can form rapidly. Disease can lead to decay and then a cycle of negative or health damaging events.

T'ai Chi Diet, Ch'ang Ming or Zhangming, can simply help you to understanding what it is you are consuming, how it relates in terms of balance and body function, and how to restore balance if your diet is less than healthy. With the never-ending onslaught of highly processed foods, junk foods and artificially produced foods that are saturating the high street eateries or supermarket shelves nowadays, that means probably 70-85% of what is purchased every day!

All you need to do is BE AWARE and make subtle changes to your diet, one by one. I will restrain myself from saying, "It really is that simple" because we have a long way to go as yet persuading governments, manufacturers and food producers to improve the countries, the industries, transport and quality of food and life in general. That is the hard part as you are fighting the many capitalist's blinkered minds.

In fact, in 2020 through 2021 we can see how the Manufacturers and big Pharmaceutical companies, backed by people like Bill Gates, are trying to push potentially dangerous mNRA vaccinations to the whole world, then make it a regular occurrence, accompanied by having your ID and Medical Records indelibly dyed into your arm. The consequences of this is to alter Genes, override the natural Immune system and create a Pharma-lead society that is totally dependent on their drugs and vaccines, at all costs: many people have died or suffered horrific health issues, but they have been stopped d from speaking as their posts have been removed by the likes of Facebook and YouTube (an estimated 200,000 victims). Any experts that posted their concerns were automatically, by a computer algorithm, labelled as "fake info' or 'false info' within one second of posting, claiming falsely that the information was read and verified by experts! This just goes to show to what extent these outrageously insane people will go to make money, and how they have no value of human lives except to use them to make more money.

Make money by all means, just make it in a healthier way and being kinder to humans and the environment!

Studying the lists below should help you to discover how you can balance your meals out so that you eat FIVE PARTS YIN to ONE PART YANG in each meal.

Yin and Yang Table of Daily Foods.

KEY: +++ Very Yang, ++ Moderate Yang, + Lesser Yang.
- - - Very Yin, - - Moderate Yin, - Lesser Yin.

FRUITS & NUTS:
- - -   Banana, Pineapple, Papaya, Mango, Grapefruit, Orange, Grapes, Dates, Figs, Pears, Pecans, Walnuts.
- -   Apricots, Lemon, Peanuts, Cashews, Almonds, Peaches, Plums, Lime, Pear, Avocado.
-   Coconut, Currants, Blueberries, Melon, Olive, Hazel-nut.
+++   None common.
++   Chestnut, Apples.
+   Strawberries, Cherry (sour red), Raspberries.

DAIRY FOODS:
- - -   Yoghurt, Cream (and Sour), Cream Cheese, Butter, Whole Cheese.
- -   Whole Cows Milk, Camembert.
-   Gruyère, Edam, Roquefort, Half Fat Cheese, Skimmed Milk.
+++   None common.
++   Goat's Cheese, Goat's Milk.
+   Dutch 'Edam' Cheese.

VEGETABLES:
- - -   Artichoke, Asparagus, Bean Sprouts, Broccoli, Cucumber, Aubergine (Egg Plant), Tomato, Yam, Potato, Mushrooms.
- -   Green Peas, Red Cabbage, Rhubarb, Squash, Celery, Lentil, Sweet Corn, Cauliflower, Brussels Sprouts, Green Peppers.
–   Green Cabbage, Bamboo Shoots, Chard, Chicory, Leeks, Beetroot, Lettuce, Sprouted Wheat.

+++ Burdock Root.
++ Pumpkin, Kale, Carrots, Dandelion (leaf), Lotus Root, Water Cress.
+   Turnip, Onion, Radish, Garlic, Beetroot, Mustard, Ginger Root.

CEREALS:
- - -   None common.
- -   None common.
-   Barley, Cornmeal (de germinated & un enriched), Oats, Rye (Whole).

+++ None common.
++   Buckwheat.
+   Brown Rice , Millet, Whole Wheat, Wheat Germ.

BEANS (PULSES):
- - - Black Beans, Chickpeas, Kidney Beans, Lima Beans, Soy Beans, String Beans, Broad Beans.
- -   Lentils, Split Peas.
-     Aduki Beans.
+++ None common.
++   None common.
+   None common.

DRINKS:
- - - Soft Drinks ('pop', 'cola', etc.), Tea (with dyes), Sparkling Wine/Champagne, Coffee (Caffeine), Chocolate, Fruit Juice.
- -   Wine, Beer, Soda.
–   Mineral Water, Deep Well/Spring Water, Herb Tea (most).

+++ Ginseng Tea (Root or Strong Extract).
++   Mu Tea, Kuzu, Umeboshi Juice.
+   Green Tea, Cocoa, Chicory, Dandelion Coffee, Yannoh.

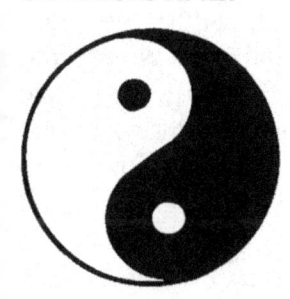

OCCASIONAL:
- - - Honey, Jam, Lard (Animal Fat), Vegetable Fat.
- -   Vegetable Oils, Soy bean Milk, Tamari.
–   Sunflower Oil/Margarine, Safflower Oil, Sesame Seeds.

+++ Seaweed, Curry Powder, Ginseng.
++   None common.
+   Human Milk, Miso, Sesame Oil, Egg.

We now have readily available cartons of Alternative Milk drinks in our shops, such as Soya, Almond and Hazelnut.

Bear in mind that Soya is generally high in unsaturated fats, and nuts are generally very high in protein. Almonds are the "fattiest" nuts, so I would highly recommend that you do a close comparison of the Per Fluid Oz or Per Serving labels on the cartons to compare fat, saturated fat, salt/sodium or potassium, etcetera. There are too many variants to be listed here.

With some modern 'healthy eating' or pre packed quick meals, you will have to buy a book on Additives (Collins Mini Gems). But generally, if you can prepare your own foods from good, wholesome fresh and natural ingredients, then you should not have any problems in maintaining a healthy body and a more worry-free life. If you really do not have the time to buy and use all fresh, local produce and resort to using tinned or pre packed, then be very careful of what you choose, mix it well with 'balancing' ingredients and remember... 'You are what you eat!'[1]

Zen and the Art of Life Maintenance.

In the earlier part of this chapter we covered the concise Taoist list of dietary dos and don'ts. You may notice that it seemed rather severe in its admonition of what appears to be most people's staple diet. Sugary drinks, meat and animal fats, processed foods and unnatural foods are definitely O-U-T! So too were an excess of spicy foods, including excess curry and pickles. Here, between the Taoist and the Zen philosophy there is a difference of opinion. Zen Monks have been known to enjoy the odd pickled radish, in moderation, of course. There is one major agreement area in all schools of thought, and this is far greater than all small differences put together - balance. The consumption of nutrients of the right type, those most compatible with the human body processes, must be consumed within the right quantities to maintain good health. Rice, wheat, millet, buckwheat and barley are the oriental staples. Just one handful of short grain brown rice, complete with its outer-shell (unpolished) contains many of the minerals, vitamins, proteins and lipids necessary to the nutrition of the human body.

De-tox Plan.

Take a handful (enough to fill the cupped palm) of Short Grain brown rice. Wash it thoroughly in cold water and then chew each mouthful until it is merely a paste. Try this as a diet for five to ten days and leave out all other food. Eat one handful of short grain brown rice early in the morning. Drink pure water only as and when you need it. If you try this detoxification plan you will purge the intestines of parasitic bacteria and give the system a chance to get rid of the toxins and other waste matter that accumulates. After just a few days you will be really amazed at the

---

[1] Brown Rice is considered to be the most perfectly balanced food as it is one part Yang to five parts Yin. White rice has little nutritional value as its best assets have been removed.

results. When this basic regime has been adhered to and you feel 100% better, then you can start adding vegetables. These should be organic, locally grown and balanced against the grain staple. The quantity should be 10% vegetables, 90% grain. Buckwheat is the most Yang grain, (and very delicious!) followed by rice, wheat and millet. Corn is the most Yin followed by rye, barley and oats. Most vegetables are quite Yin, especially after cooking or processing. Romaine lettuce, radishes, onions, parsley, tofu, Chinese cabbage, watercress, turnip, kale and carrots are some of the Yang ones. But do not forget, the proportion should be five parts Yin to one part Yang. If you do not adhere carefully to this dietary balance then you will end up being really Sanpaku again. One of the most noticeable effects of following the plan is that after you have cleansed the system your brain becomes sharper and you may also experience more 'ESP' type occurrences. Do not be alarmed. The human mind is capable of many things and if you think about it, there is little difference between physically hearing and translating another person's voice and mentally putting out or receiving other communication signals (thoughts or feelings). All forms of thought are like radio waves and the brain a transmitter/receiver.

There is a theory that runs among most practitioners of the old Oriental Arts. It says that in this day and age, influenced by strong Western culture that we are poisoning ourselves, falling prey to the bilge and bull of the advertising media. Men and women are becoming de-sexed through what they eat and the way they are educated in mixed classes (they emulate each other). This leads to 'women-men' and 'men-women', as one person aptly described it. We are what we eat and if we eat lots of Yin food then we become Yin people. If we eat lots of Yang food, likewise we become overly Yang. An adversely affected man or woman's attitude becomes more selfish, arrogant or aggressive, society becomes possessed by the 'Me!' and 'I WANT...!' syndrome, relationships and sex-lives are damaged, our families and friends bear the brunt of the whims and moods, and those who suffer try to convince others that they alone are 'normal'. Cancer, leukaemia, leucorrhoea and the like would not be so common if we could all only get back to a sensible diet. It is not just the consumption of meat that is to blame for our lot. It is all the atmospheric pollution (mainly industrial) food additives, processing and unnecessary altering of basics, as well as the imbalance of Yin/Yang, that accounts for much of the illnesses we suffer. If we look at Great Britain the figures show that the British have the sweetest tooth in Europe. Is it surprising as most infants are weaned on foods that have refined sugar added, often in high quantities?

In Zen and Tibetan Buddhism animal flesh is forbidden for good reason. Animal flesh is all right for animals that are naturally equipped to hunt, kill and devour their prey. For this purpose they have a different kind of digestive system. Sugar is available in the forms of sucrose, fructose and glucose in the natural fruits and vegetables that we consume; we really do not need to eat artificially produced sugars. Humans have the potential to be able to develop their thinking along higher paths, eventually obtaining peace and wisdom. This cannot be done when the system is clogged-up with cholesterol and acids, toxins and other unwanted waste. However, if enlightenment does not mean that much to you then adjust gradually over the course of a few years. Anyone who practises, worse still teaches, any form of so-called enlightenment exercise and eats meat and artificial 'junk food' is just playing on a drum with no skin!

This gives you a gentle insight into the Yin and Yang of foods. There is, of course, much more to it than this. Your diet is something which should never be neglected and has to be studied over a period of time. However, a long time master of the T'ai Chi of Diet may be well equipped to cope naturally and gracefully with daily changes and conditions. In the olden days of China's history, doctors were paid as long as you were well and healthy. As soon as one's health deteriorated in any way the payments stopped until a cure was found! However, this was only good for those who could afford to pay the doctor his fees, especially for large families in poorer areas. Thus there have always been many divisions in medicine but only one has ever remained number one in the list of importance - the ability to prevent disease or illness by living correctly. I leave you with a famous saying. 'Physician, heal thyself!'

Personal Enquiry.
What makes us eat what we do, for example, why do we eat meat, is it because of old wives' tales, like "meat makes you strong", just because you like the taste - e.g. salty bacon, or what?

A Doctor's Independent Review.

Milton M. Mills, M.D., (USA) did some very thorough and unbiased studies on the gastrointestinal tracts and processes of humans and other animals.

He says that he did this because he got rather tired of patients asking "What should I eat?" Or arguing for or against meat, etcetera. He decided that the only way to resolve this issue was to do a professional research into the digestive systems of animals and humans, then publish the results.

His conclusion. "In conclusion, we see that human beings have the gastrointestinal tract structure of a 'committed' herbivore. Humankind does not show the mixed structural features one expects and finds that in anatomical omnivores such as bears and raccoons. Thus, from comparing the gastrointestinal tract [and mastication system] of humans to that of carnivores, herbivores and omnivores we must conclude that humankind's GI tract is designed for a purely plant-food diet."

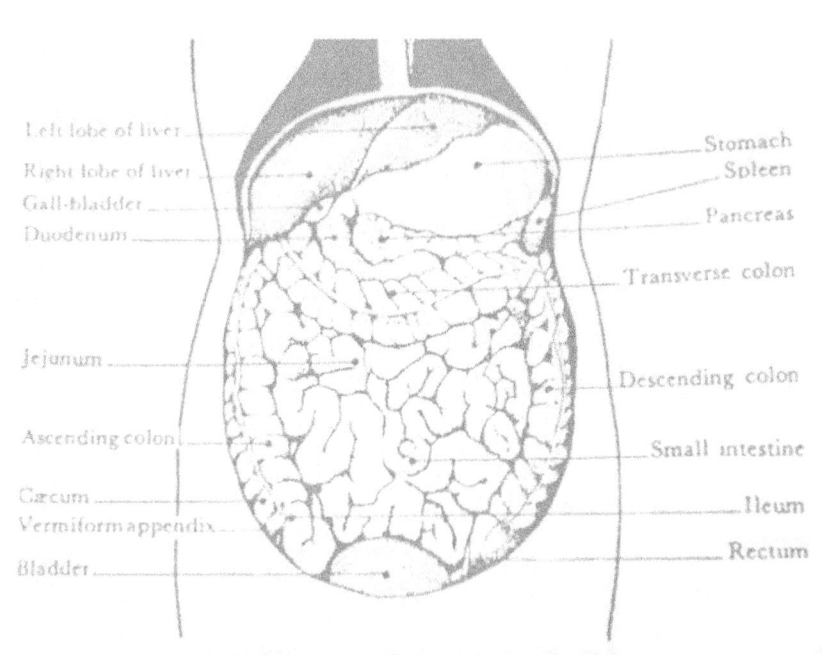

THE ORGANS OF DIGESTION, ETC.

THE FIVE ELEMENTS

The Five Elements (Wu Hsing) are the real key to the Chinese Dietary System, T'ai Chi Ch'uan (Taiji Quan), Ch'uan-shu (Quan-zu or "Kung-fu" - slang) and Traditional Chinese Medicine (TCM). The Five Elements are the next evolution from the Yin and Yang and they describe the basic principles of creation, destruction and interaction, which give rise to all things. To describe to you the basic composition of the Five Elements is one thing, but the minds that first studied the workings of the Universe and equated them with such a simplistic yet wholesome science for the people is something to ponder.

The ancient Taoist sages of China 'observed'. They observed and compared notes, studied and learned and then observed more. Very scientific. Perhaps in the West our educational system encourages us to "complete the Uni course", after which we are told that it is done and that we can go out and use "it" (whatever the knowledge or subject is). This concept simply does not exist in the Taoist Arts and the basic principle that governed the ancient ways in China was, 'if it works use it and if you feel enthused by it then study and learn, develop and teach'. This is why the Taoist Arts cover so much ground.

What may be beyond most people's comprehension, at first, is the fact that the Taoist philosophy with its symbolic concepts of Yin/Yang, Wu Hsing and Pa Kua (Eight Diagrams or Directions; as used in the 'I Ching' book) is the prevalent hub of so many Arts. From Almanac to Food, Horoscopes to Ch'uan-shu, healing to yoga and strategy to Zen (Ch'an). The involvements can be seen everywhere, naturally. Nature and her actions and interactions may be observed and the wise attempt to flow with her.

After Yin/Yang, the two basic forces of the Universe, or Multiverses, the next separation in terms of distinction are the Five Elements.

Note: If you are a student, studying health, Traditional Chinese Medicine, or even just Balanced Nutrition, then it will be important for you to understand these correlations in Elements and Yin/Yang. Anyone concerned about improving their diet might also benefit from "getting the idea" as understanding The Five Elements and The Five Flavours is an important part of balancing your own health (see the Table below).

The Five Elements are; Water, Wood, Fire, Earth, Metal.
Each of these has a Yin or a Yang side. Each can be 'creative' or 'destructive' or balanced against the others. In the case of diet the observations relate to how one type of food may cause problems if not balanced by another. These effects may be compounded by the Elemental effects of the seasons, one's personal elements by birth-time and the environments in which you work and live. Now you begin to appreciate just how deep this "simple" science is! The Wu Hsing are not separate from the Yin and Yang, but an extension of it, like branches of a Family Tree.

What I call "Forwards Trace" enables us to understand the flow of the Universe or its parts, so from Yin we trace through to Still, Passive, Negative and Water to reach "Stagnation". In "Backwards Trace" we can name the effect that caused the stagnation we see; Stagnation is caused by too much Yin or inactivity.

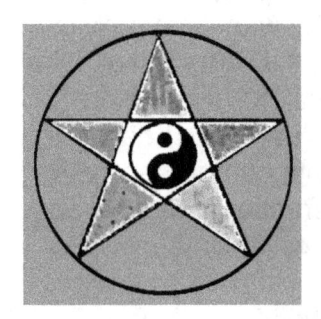

WU HSING

The Wu Hsing (Five Elements) theory are used to link the internal organs and functions with their associated health or disease properties in a similar simplistic manner. There are two cycles, *destructive* (Yin) and *creative* (Yang): Creative is helping better health while Destructive is Pathogens and illness. Within this pattern the Five Yang and the Five Yin organs are associated with Five Elements;

YIN VISCERA - ORGANS

CREATIVE CYCLE (YANG)
(The Five Viscera) Heart = Fire, Spleen = Earth, Lungs = Metal, Kidneys = Water and Liver = Wood.

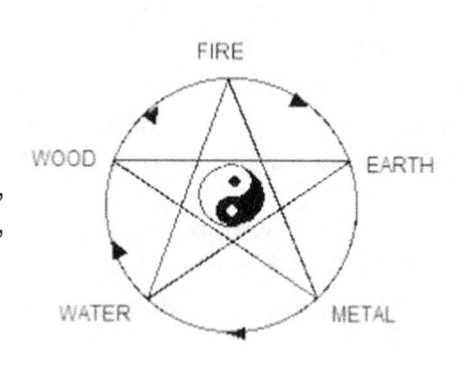

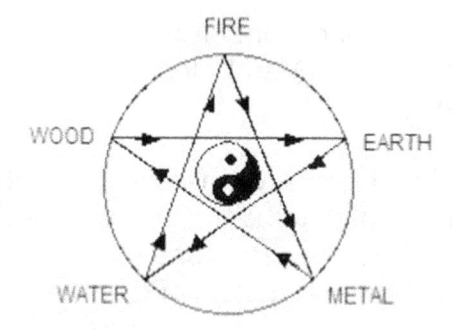

YANG VISCERA 'BOWELS'

DESTRUCTIVE CYCLE (YIN)
(The Five Bowels) Small Intestine = Fire, Large Intestine = Metal, Gallbladder = Wood, Stomach = Earth and Bladder = Water.

Thus we are left with the simple to follow theory that in the destructive cycle the element of Fire, in excess, will destroy Metal. In terms of illness this would mean that as the 'Heart' relates to the emotions, an excess of emotions (stress, anxiety, grief, etcetera) could lead to skin ailments (lung/large intestine and body tissues) such as eczema, allergy and also to such common problems as stress related asthma. Should the condition of the Lung Meridians and associated organs worsen then the 'knock-on' effect is to the liver/gallbladder, for fire controls metal and metal controls wood. There would be several ways to treat this problem, once it had been correctly diagnosed. Acupressure or acupuncture will have an almost immediate effect on the flow of the bioenergy and can relieve symptoms quite quickly. It also may redress the balance after one or several treatments, depending on the exact nature of the problem and its intensity. Herbal remedies may be useful in supplying counter agents to produce the desired relief or partial recovery. Ch'i Kung (Qigong) exercises may be given to either stimulate the flow of the bioenergy or more physical exercises recommended to promote the strength of the tissues, organs or functions in particular areas. Diet is another important aspect. To strengthen the lungs, for our example above, we would need to consume more 'earthy' foods; millet, dates and olives, chicken (organic), and thyme as a herbal drink. To strengthen the heart and calm the emotions we would need to ruminate more 'woody' foods; wheat, leeks, apples and ginseng. Thus we would be strengthening the organs via the creative cycle.

The basic descriptions of the 'creative cycle' are that Water (liquid) creates Wood (Growth) and Wood creates Fire (Heat or Energy), Fire creates Earth (Soil, Minerals, Metals) and from this we come to Water again.

The basics of the 'destructive cycle' (also called 'controlling cycle') are that Water puts out Fire, Fire controls Metal, Metal cleaves Wood, Wood cleaves Earth and Earth dampens Fire.

To understand how this relates to food and health we need to think of each element in broader terms. So Fire relates to heat, energy, fever, redness, sweating, laughing and irritability (as in a rash or discomfort). As stated earlier, not everything is necessarily in a state of creation or destruction, though there will be fluxes one way or the other with everyone. Understanding these relationships helps us to a) know ourselves and our world, b) to adjust our daily environment and diet, plus c) recognise imbalance and restore balance. Thus we achieve 'Harmony'. This applies not just to foods but to relationships and everything else.

If the Five Elements are not in harmony then we feel the effects in whatever way the imbalance relates to. The number Five also describes many 'sections' or divisions, seasons, tastes, smells and colours. The table which follows is a full composition of the Taoist Elemental Relationships of Health; often referred to in other books but rarely seen in this its complete form. My Master passed this knowledge on to me and I pass it on to you so that you may learn it, learn from it and in turn pass it on as you help others. Use it as a reference when trying to understand an illness or imbalance; some imbalances you may not "see" until you have studied the references, for there are many imbalances that we take for granted in every day life. Study and observe.

This gives you more knowledge about the action and interaction of foods, their balance and effect on the human body. These principles are used in TCM for diagnostics and treatments: e.g. simply put, someone on a too Yin diet will be recommended a bit more Yang foods to address the imbalance.

In an earlier chapter I dealt with diagnostics by colour recognition. This is taken further and linked to the Five Yin organs and the Five Yang organs. Each organ has an Element to represent it that suitably relates to the others in term of 'creative' or 'destructive' actions. The liver (wood) leads on to the heart (fire), this leads on beneficially to the spleen (earth) and this to the lungs (metal) which leads on to the kidneys (water). One organ draws energy from another so that, as in nature, each element serves the next. We can examine it another way. The liver (wood) passes energy to the muscles, which helps us develop a strong heart (fire). The heart (fire) enables nourishment to be passed via the blood to the Spleen (earth) which nurtures the flesh (metal) and strengthens the lungs (metal). The lungs (metal) then feed the skin (tissues) with oxygen from which we draw other energies and this boosts the kidneys (water) which relates to enhancements of the liver.

From this it is said that:

1) The liver is in charge of the muscles and tissue.
2) The heart is in charge of the arteries and body texture.
3) The spleen is in charge of the flesh (including lips).
4) The lungs are in charge of the skin and hair.
5) The kidneys are in charge of the bones and nails.

Whilst this may not make immediate Orthodox medical sense, further studies reveal more depth. In general terms this is called the 'Mother and Child Relationship': Taken literally, if a mother breast feeds her baby and the milk is not of the right quality then the baby will be affected; just as pregnant women who smoke or take any drugs will pass on those harmful things in her bloodstream to the baby. Conversely, if the milk is not nutritious enough then the baby will not feel satisfied and will want to continue drawing from the mother. This will have the effect of depleting the mother's energy and her becoming ill and unable to support the child. Each organ, if depleted, will draw on the next and eventually all the organs will be depleted and illness sets in. Hence the Mother and Child Relationship in TCM sees the effect of one organ or function, when in disharmony, as influencing the next one, and so on.

TCM principles use a different approach to those of Western Medicine and it would be near enough impossible to draw any comparisons between the major and minor organs, bodily functions and relationships the way that TCM and Orthodox Medicine see them. What the following chart does is to link the important organs with the fundamental substances and activities; storing/spreading, absorbing/eliminating, ascending/descending, preserving/transforming and so on. It follows the well developed TCM theories and links certain 'conditions' with corresponding states; this having been achieved at great length over hundreds of years by strict observations.

According to the Mother and Child relationship, if a person is suffering from a condition of the spleen and pancreas, then there will be troubles with the stomach and late summer would be the worst time as would the daily periods of afternoon. They should stay away from the equator region and avoid humidity. The skin may take on a yellow hue beneath the surface and there may be a tendency to sing spontaneously. The quality of the flesh will be poor and there will be tell-tale signs in the lips and tongue. The cure will be a mixture of Herbal Therapy (ginseng and ginger are beneficial), eating millet, black dates, olives and apricots, whilst avoiding raw foods (general Western type salads, unless "warmed" with ginger dressing) and thyme tea. An imbalance in one organ, as previously stated, will drain from the organ that comes before it in the cycle of control and deprive the organ after it. Thus eventually all five organs become depleted; the Five Yin Viscera multiplied by the Five Elements gives us twenty-five types of disharmony. If the illness is not checked, and then becomes worse, the Yin organs start to draw energy from the Five Yang organs, which produces another five times five, equalling another twenty-five disharmonies. Eventually the twenty-five multiplies by twenty-five to give us six-hundred-and-twenty-five disharmonies. When there are that many problems in the body things are radically wrong and serious illness sets in. Illnesses such as advanced cancer are representative of this stage. How can Western Physicians hope to cure cancer by looking at *it* alone? Cancer, like any other illness, takes place as part of a complete system and is not a separate entity. Traditional Chinese Medicine looks at the body, its environment, intake, output (skin colouring, urine, excrement quality, skin conditions, etcetera) as a rightful whole. Therefore, with any illness, it is vital to see your nearest Ch'ang Ming consultant and correct the imbalance before anything serious illness is allowed to develop. In the course of my days I see many people, ranging from students of 'Kung-fu' or Taiji and Qigong to people I know and like, who work in local shops or public houses where I may go for a drink occasionally. Here are some examples:

CASE HISTORIES.
(Case 1) Miss 'L'. She is lively, lovely and gregarious with a loving nature and outgoing personality. She suffers from asthma and this is indicated by her 'white' complexion. She worked in a smoky public house. She has almost constant back aches, large intestine troubles and spasmodic painful periods. This is the lung problem drawing from the spleen/pancreas. Help and advice was offered by myself to her of Acupressure and dietary advice; at no charge and simply because, like other Taoist Arts Masters I care, and it is not good to see decent people suffering. Some advice was taken, but not enough due to being 'too busy'. So far, this 'Horse' has been led to water but is not drinking; again, this Western attitude towards accepting illness and doing nothing about it instead of accepting good health and rejecting illness.

(Case 2) Mr 'A', an ex-student of Taoist Quan-shu. Works in a bakery where there is no adequate ventilation and ever present dust, powders and fumes in the air and does not wear a breathing mask. Not surprisingly he complains of a tight chest. Although he has slightly darker skin, the underlying colour is white. Dryness (Heat & Dust) is the climatic or environmental condition that should be avoided (his working conditions) and the air should be humidified. His energy will be affected as the spleen/pancreas is drawn from and this provides the necessary balance between blood sugar levels. Weeping (overproduction of fluids from the eyes) may be experienced and therefore more mucus from the nose*. In his case I would recommend that he somehow humidifies the air and includes the appropriate foods, herbs and drinks in his diet. Again, there is no charge for my time or advice.

* A condition which may also come from Fan heating, such as that found in Night Storage radiators.

If you just look around you at all the people you know who have this underlying white complexion and they all are prone to colds, influenza, asthma and general sinus troubles. The Ch'ang Ming (Long Life Diet) recommendations for part of the cure are; brown rice, onions, anything containing mustard oil, peaches, apricots, melons, milk, rabbit or hare if they are meat eaters, fruit juice and beer. They must avoid rotten foods and anything pungent (spicy or tangy). To strengthen the spleen a little millet, black dates and herbal therapy can be applied. Of course, this merely written information excludes by that fact treatments including Acupressure or acupuncture and follow on diagnostics to detect any change or further needs of treatments. However, this section gives you enough insight into the Chinese Art of recognising imbalances.

The idea for obtaining balance is to correct any imbalances by using the above diagnostic methods and 'restore' the strength of the organ that is affected. After treating one organ there may another to restore; by using the controlling cycle you will see which. As with Homeopathy, treating varied levels or separate illnesses is like peeling back the layers of an onion until you come to the core; this being the last stage. Once everything has been treated and there are no underlying colours or other indications of imbalance, then you can concentrate on eating the right balance of foods and doing balanced things in your life or balancing your environment. This may be done by using the chart above with the earlier tables of Yin or Yang Foodstuffs (observe the Greater Yin, Lesser Yin, Yin/Yang or "balanced", Lesser Yang and greater Yang principles and place the foods appropriately in each category). In harmony the healthy liver passes on its energy to help the heart. If the heart is getting the right foods then it will in turn pass on its energy to the spleen/pancreas, and so on. Thus a healthy person maintains balance by preventing illness and small "wobbles" may be detected and prevented from developing into an illness at an early stage.

SUMMARY

Because of the ignorance about health in the West I often feel that half the people with whom I come into casual contact with do not take me seriously. It is truly frustrating to have this knowledge and information at your fingertips, to be able to see, recognise and diagnose problems with people that you know or meet and yet be able to do nothing about it. Westerners, and even many of those from the East nowadays, are ignorant of the facts. Orthodox practitioners (midwives, hospitals, family doctors, etc.) have brought about a system whereby people are taught to rely upon them from an early age; it starts with prenatal care and personally at infancy. This could be the problem as people are brought up to rely on someone else for their problems when the real onus should be upon themselves. Methods of diagnostics between East and West are about as far apart as can be. From a logical point of view I cannot see the need for those who get illness to pump drugs and chemicals into their body and cause possible further damage by doing so. It just does not make sense to me, especially when I have personal knowledge of a system whereby one can detect imbalance at an early stage and using advanced diagnostic systems, which do not need equipment, make changes for the better by adjusting one's diet, or exercise. Further to this we can add Moxibustion and Herbal treatments, Energy Training (Qigong), Acupressure (Dian Xue) and Acupuncture, Tui Na (massage and manipulation) and general massage (An Mo), External Qi Healing (Wai Qi Liao Fa) and even environmental significant or Feng Shui (Pron. "Fung Sho-way").

My old Taoist Arts Master was a man of immense knowledge; he was a teacher and a healer. It is with honour that I attempt to follow in his footsteps and both teach and practice what he passed on to me. In order to achieve this, books like these are needed as it seems the Western public would, generally, rather read it at leisure than hear it or experience it first hand. Also the Taoist principle of giving freely is a concept that capitalist societies cannot grasp too well. There are some of his students who are carrying on his traditional Li or 'Lee' Family Arts and it is a pleasure to announce that his books are being reproduced (look for books by Chee Soo) and should be of interest perhaps to anyone reading this book and studying Taoist Arts or Chinese Arts and philosophy in general.

The chapters of this book, and especially the key chapter above, will help you to understand, but more importantly, *recognise* for yourself what ails you or what is below par in your loved ones. Not that I am recommending you all take to becoming an instant physician overnight! As I intimated above, it is about self-awareness and lifestyles. In the theory of TCM the first and foremost element in the chain of problems and treatments is that of looking after yourself and avoiding illness.

Below, on the next page, is the Five Element Theory Table. This shows in simple layout the relationship between the diagnostics, conditions and their repair using balanced foods (meat is shown here but not necessarily advocated).

This chart may be of more interest to practitioners of TCM or dieticians. It represents hundreds, if not thousands of years of scientific study (even though it might not have been called 'science' originally) by thousands of people who collated their information and then formalised it into this chart.

This book can serve as a ready guide to many common problems which are brought about by imbalanced diets. Those problems caused by regular consumption of "junk foods", unnatural and processed foods, such as found in many chain outlets across the globe, may be much harder to work on and take more years, as long as the damage has not become irreparable.
    It is also meant a lasting learning guide to the precious Taoist Ch'ang Ming Dietary skills that have taken so many years to be researched and developed. The longest standing health and life skills on the planet. These must never be lost.

Parents.
Heads up, pay attention please. Children really are not suited to making their own choices. You, the responsible guardian, need to understand the problems they are about to encounter and give practical advice in a calm and factual manner. Explain the differences, the outcomes, then tell them that you are doing this for them because you love them and do not want to see them suffer in later life. Be warned though, the advertisements are powered by psychology, in words and colours, even playing on parental issues, like "Aww, I let my kids have a treat at Big Mucky because they love it so much!" You are fighting a battle, not only for your children but for yourselves.

Don't Just Read, Study.
It may need long and careful study of the rest of this book, and possibly others, before becoming clearer to you. I will apologise now for the quality of the following chart as I produced it in an old PC program and converted it into a table graphics, hence it has lost some quality, but for all intents and purposes it is still readable. Producing a big book such as this requires many, many months, using too many different PC Programmes and, of course, years of study and research beforehand.

The Five Element Theory of Food & Ailment Diagnostic Table

	The Five Elements				
	Greater Yang:	Lesser Yang:	Yang/Yin:	Lesser Yin:	Greater Yin:
Wu Hsing:	Wood	Fire	Earth	Metal	Water
Viscera	Liver	Heart	Spleen/Pancr's	Lungs	Kidneys
Bowels	Gall Bladder	Sm. Intestine	Stomach	Lg. Intestine	Bladder
Seasons	Spring	Summer	Late Summer	Autumn	Winter
Daily Periods	Morning	Noon	Afternoon	Evening	Night
Planets	Jupiter	Mars	Saturn	Venus	Mercury
Directions	East	South	Equator	West	North
Weather	Dry/Crisp	Fog/Mist	Mellow	Snow	Frost/Ice
Colours	Green	Red	Yellow	White	Black
Climatic Conditions	Wind	Heat	Humidity	Dryness	Cold
Influence	Spirit	Soul	Mind	Ambition	Phy. Strength
Creation	Inspiration	Aspiration	Intellect	Dominance	Will
Emotions	Shouting	Laughing	Singing	Weeping	Groaning
Fluids	Tears	Sweat	Saliva	Mucus	Urine
Anatomy (Int)	Muscles	Arteries	Flesh	Skin	Bones
Anatomy (Ext)	Tissues	Complexion	Lips	Hair	Nails
Senses	Sight	Hearing	Taste	Smell	Touch
Openings	Eyes	Ears	Mouth	Nose	Lower Cavities
Mental Stress	Anger	Joy	Sympathy	Grief	Fear
Sickness	Nerves	Viscera	Tongue	Back	Cavities
Best Cure	Spiritual	Ch'ang Ming	Herbal Therapy	Acupuncture	Thermogenisis
Ideal food	Wheat	Corn	Millet	Rice	Peas/beans
Vegetables	Leeks	Shallots	Mallow	Onions	Coarse Greens
Fruit	Apples	Strawberry & Cherry	Dates & Olives	Peaches & Melons	Grapefruit & Oranges
Animal Foods	Pheasants Egg Yolks	Turkey & Pigeon	Chicken	Rabbit & Hare	Pork & Beef
Dairy Foods	Goat's Milk	Vege'n Cheese	Edam Cheese	Milk	Butter/Yoghurt
Drinks or Herbs	Ginseng	Mugwort & Fo Ti Tien	Thyme	Fruit Juice or Beer	Coffee & Tea
Liking For	Sour	Bitter	Sweet	Pungent	Salty
Avoid these	Rancid	Overdone	Fragrant	Rotten	Putrid

Author's Note: This Table was created in a Spreadsheet Program but has lost some quality in being converted into a usable image. However, it still serves as a perfectly usable example of the Five Element Relationships. Study this, or come back to it, regularly, and it will gradually become more clear to you.

BASIC FOOD PROPERTIES

Among the most common errors of diet is the tendency to eat too much sweet foodstuff, much of which is artificial (e.g.; boiled sweets, toffee, etcetera.) and made from beet sugar; also totally unnatural! As you will see below in the chapter on Nutrition, there are many different properties that we need to maintain a healthy and positive life. The most common foods eaten by humans around the world are those of a leafy, root or fruit type (berries, seeds, nuts, and anything which has seeds). These form by far the largest part of most people's diets in most countries. We get essential vitamins and minerals from a variety of plants and products, but the amounts we get vary according to where we live. The quality of the soil, even from state to state or county to county, will affect the overall quality of the foods grown in that area. Even locally the soil may have a different value to that which is just twenty kilometres away. This is why farmers, in the more affluent parts of the world, constantly test the quality of their soil and add lime, phosphorus, blood or bone meal (from slaughter houses) or other elements as needed. Organic farmers will only use natural fertilisers. Obviously, if this concerns you and you are curious about the quality of the food you eat, then you need to research your own case; Where do you buy your food from? Where does the shop/market stall/supermarket get it from? Where was it grown or produced and under what conditions: e.g. is it organic? What is the status of the soil in that area?

In this day and age it is particularly difficult to know exactly what we are eating. Even though technology has progressed to a point where we can test the qualities of just about anything, we cannot get reliable information about the status of our comestibles. On the side of many packets are details about the average contents; vitamins, minerals, trace elements and energy. These figures are only averages though. What we want to know as well is; what is the origin? How old is it? How many vitamins will be left by the time we actually get around to preparing it and eating it? (Vitamins begin losing potency as soon as a plant/fruit is picked, the longer we keep it, the more it loses. Cooking will also destroy much vitamin content). Is it grown organically and untreated after harvesting? Does the farmer use animal by-products on his land (e.g.; blood & bone meal)? What effects does the packaging have on us? (Recent tests show that cling film, certain plastics, tin linings and other items can seriously affect our health).

The chart below will give you some ideas as to the best sources of our essential vitamins and the processes for which they are required. Eating correctly is something of a science, but only a simple science. It need not be too much of a chore to work out our best course of action in planning a healthier diet.

The common sense approach is to start with one thing at a time; cut out one bad food, then add one better food to your diet. Get used to the idea of what that food is doing for you. When you realise that it makes you feel better then you will soon be willing to learn about another foodstuff and what it does for you. Gradually you will change your life from one of constant illness to one of better energy and more enjoyment. Most people make the mistake of trying to change everything at once, and not many of us can do that; I certainly could not, but one step at a time I found much easier. After having been a vegetarian since 1970, I now find that I am fitter and stronger than ever I was as a teenager or young man. The practice of Taoist Ch'uan-shu (Wudang Quanshu) and T'ai Chi Ch'uan (Taijiquan) certainly work hand-in-hand with this and apart from one or two tell-tale signs of body abuse when I was younger, everything works exceedingly well. Even those who hate exercise must face the fact that the body needs exercise to stay healthy, process foods, grow new skin, bone, etcetera. What I love about the Taoist or Wudang Arts is that they are holistic, including health and diet, healing and self-defence with mind-expanding philosophy that applies to all things in the Universe.

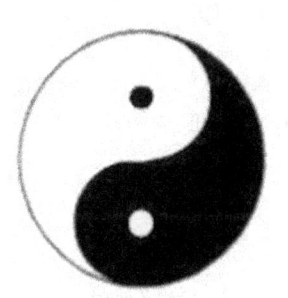

Yang & Yin

The two major forces of the Universe.
Neither is one-hundred percent but contains the seed of the other.
Yang, because it represents action, change, force and growth,
it needs comparably larger amounts of Yin to counteract it:
hence in Ch'ang Ming we eat 3 parts Yin to 2 parts Yang.

NOTE: Always stick as close as you can to your recommended daily allowance. This can be determined from a chart usually printed on the labels of dietary supplement packages, such as multi-vitamins. Take into account that most prepared foods have added vitamin and mineral contents; mainly A, C, D and B12 with some containing Iron, which is good: e.g. Spreads, breakfast cereals, children's drinks/snacks, etc.

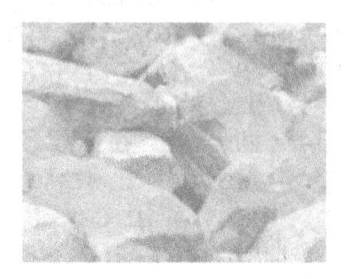

MINERALS: (See 'Minerals and their functions' below.) Those which act as constituents of the body tissues include; Phosphorus, zinc, sulphur, iron and copper - present in muscle, blood corpuscles, the liver or special structures.

Those that are soluble salts, maintaining consistency of body fluids; Sodium, chlorine and potassium.

Those which are needed for the skeletal structure; Calcium, phosphorus, fluorine and magnesium.

Others needed in regulated doses; Iodine, copper, manganese, cobalt (See B12), salt (sodium chloride). Others in minute 'trace' quantities.

Iron-rich foods: Oatmeal, wholemeal flour and bread; lentils, haricot beans and dried peas; dried apricots, dried figs, prunes, raisins and blackcurrants; eggs; spinach, green peas, broccoli, water cress, cabbage.

Body-building foods: Eggs, dried peas and beans (legumes). Also milk and cheese.

Protective foods: Vegetables, potatoes and fruit (fresh, not tinned or processed); vitamin-added margarine (sunflower or other low in saturated fats), Nuts, (fresh) Fruits.

Protein Rich Foods: Beans & Legumes (10-35% by weight), Corn (13% by weight), Flour Gluten (70%), Nuts (15-30%) Pumpkin Seeds/Sesame Seeds/Sunflower seeds (17-24%), Rice (7%).

Fuel foods: Bread, flour (including pastry, but not 'white') and whole cereals.

Immune System: (see also 'Covid' Section)
The Immune System is a combined operation and a complex yet adaptive process. It identifies harmful germs or virus and activates special cells to destroy them. After doing so it creates a "memory" of that germ/virus so as to recognise it more quickly in the future – a 'database'. The next time the offender, or one of its variant relatives enters your system, the Immune system recognises it from the database and sends out a rapid assault force to dispatch it. You may not even notice, let alone become ill.

The Immune System has to be kept healthy, this includes allowing to deal with germs, virus, etc. ("training"!) You need to eat the right foods and absorb all the right vitamins and minerals to make it work 100%. In the main, you need Vitamin D, Zinc, Magnesium, Calcium and Selenium, K2 and Vitamin C. Researchers are still discovering more about this natural function, but are starting to think that other elements may also play a role in the process, such as Copper or even B12.

As you can see by the above categories of mineral rich foods that we need for daily health, growth and repair, they can again be found in *natural* foods. This can be a problem in the so-called civilised countries, as Natural Food can be quite hard to come by! Many foods, even vegetables, are sprayed with chemicals to enhance growth and poisons to kill "pests": not really pests, just insects that live or breed on vegetation!

Eating naturally, or as naturally as possible, with fresh and organic foods is a recurring theme in this book. That is because it is one of the main guidelines in Ch'ang Ming - Taoist 'Long Life' Diet - as is the act of eating produce that is In Season and Local. If you have a garden, away from any busy roads where petrochemical residue from exhausts may contaminate, then try growing fresh vegetables and keep some hens (who will eat insects), you will be glad you did. Fresh, locally grown, organic and "just picked" foods taste absolutely superb!

Simple Rules:
- Eat as many fresh, <u>in season</u>, local, untreated foods as often as you possibly can.
- Eat three small meals per day if possible
- Always eat breakfast, the most important meal of the day.
- Try to have your main meal around or *before* midday: the digestive system is working at its peak in the Chinese Body Clock theory.
- Avoid eating heavy meals after seven p.m.
- Healthy snacks are all right in between meals if you are working very hard.
- Aid your digestion by sitting up straight. After 15 minutes go for a walk.
- Exercise regularly, but only two hours after eating meals.

The Chinese Body Clock Qi Flow Theory (as used in Acupuncture)

Liver 1 a.m. - 3 a.m.	Lung 3 a.m. - 5 a.m.
Large. Intestine 5 a.m. - 7 a.m.	Stomach 7 a.m. - 9 a.m.
Spleen 9 a.m.- 11 a.m.	Heart 11 a.m. - 1 p.m.
Small Intestine 1 p.m. - 3 p.m.	Bladder 3 p.m. - 5 p.m.
Kidney 5 p.m. - 7 p.m.	Pericardium 7 p.m. - 9 p.m.
Triple Warmer 9 p.m. - 11 p.m.	Gall Bladder 11 p.m. - 1 a.m.

The Spleen Meridian governs transportation and transformation, extracting nutrients from the stomach and transforming blood and qi. This, according to my teachers, means that you should try to eat the most important meals of the day when the qi flow dealing with the digestive processes is at its strongest.

Many people in the Westernised areas have a very small breakfast, then either go without lunch or have a small snack, then eat dinner at some time between 7 pm and 10 pm. This is why so many people put on weight and find it hard or impossible to loose. The metabolic processes slow down and the fuel which remains unused (probably around 85%) is stored as fat.

Young women who smoke their way through lunch break, or eat a small yoghurt, may find that the smoking reduces appetite. Whilst they are young the effects may not be noticed, apart from the odd dizzy attack, or feeling 'strange', but as they get older their bodies are likely to age more quickly. Seems pointless? It is. Eat sensibly: have a good breakfast, like porridge, eat a hearty lunch (this will be worked off) and then enjoy a light and healthy meal as soon as you finish work. Of course, smoking is stupid. Follow this very simple plan and live longer, look younger and feel much, much better into later life.

Important Note: Vitamin D is one of the hardest to get from daily foods, especially if you are vegetarian or Vegan, as mostly this vitamin is found in fish, and some dairy produce. Getting sunlight on your body for periods up to 20 minutes or so will enable the body to produce it's own Vitamin D, provided your diet allows. However, Skin Cancer is also a risk from the Sun's rays, especially given the weakening of the Ozone layer that used to protect us!

A good supplement should be had to make sure the Immune System is kept healthy and fully functional. Vitamin D3 is utilised more quickly than D, so should be active within a few days, whereas D will take up to 4 weeks.

The Pandemic of Covid-19 that began in November 2019 through to March 2020 - then mutated to around 30+ Variants - showed us that many, many thousands of people needlessly died who had an insufficient and unhealthy Immune System*.

Once started, take daily.

* Note: people die needlessly every year from Flu or other Covid Variants, heart disease, Cancer, organ failure and many other so-called "common illnesses". The NHS and its likenesses around the world seem to concentrate on applying drugs or surgery. Drastic measures indeed. If Preventative Medicine was established and cast broadly out into the community, many families could enjoy the company of their loved ones for much longer.

"Prevention is better than cure"
Nothing is more true than this age old saying. Prevention starts here, so understand what you eat, what you really need, and prevent many common ailments.

On the following pages we take a fairly wholesome look at Vitamins, what they are, what they do and where we can get them from. This has not been made too specific, but most people who wish to be healthy, if eating animal flesh, would start by becoming Vegetarian. Animals that are reared for slaughter are never quite "organic", as injections may be used at times for various reasons. These injections may become residue in the flesh, not intended to be consumed by people. Quite apart from that, the blood may contain bacteria which are not meant for humans but might cause illness: just look at the concerns about the Virus transfer.

While some animals have been included, such as fish, or animal by-products, such as cheese, the reader should be sensible and make his or her own choices based upon their health, conditions and medical needs, such as Diabetes, Asthma, Arthritis, etc. Some people may not be able to tolerate a 100% Vegan diet, or Vegetarian, so might become Pescetarian (Pescetarianism is the practice of using seafood as the only source of meat in a diet that is otherwise vegetarian). This may also be a stepping stone in dietary change, after all, Rome wasn't built in a day and the human body cannot change or adapt overnight.

Please be sensible about dietary changes and do not engage in trendy diets that you see advertised in magazines or on YouTube Channels. These can be very dangerous indeed, especially when advertised for "miracle weight loss". Be warned!

The author does highly recommend that you study the next section carefully, making note of any current foods compared to the daily needs, to get some idea of just how much of your diet is actually giving you of what you really need. Remember the motto of this book - List and Lose, but only one step at a time.

DAILY VITAMIN & MINERAL NEEDS

The amount of vitamins and minerals we need every day has been long established and we are all now familiar with the charts on the sides of packaged foodstuffs which state the vitamin contents and the UK's RNI (Reference Nutritional Intake) and the USA's RDA (Recommended Daily Allowance) of the vitamins and minerals in either micrograms (mcg) or milligrams (mg). The chart below will give you an indication of what you need every day as an average healthy male of 25 to 50 years, weighing approximately 174 lb (12 Stone). It will not tell you what you are actually getting. You have to work out that for yourselves by monitoring your daily input to make sure that you are not getting too little or too much.

Some RDA's come in measures of International Units (iu), RNI, micrograms (mcg) or milligrams (mg), as used here. The chart here is based on the average adult male in the U.K. or U.S.A. (not female as dietary requirements vary much according to weight, time of the month and factors such as pregnancy). See your Clinical Dietician for your personal needs at any given time.

This chart uses the newer definitions of μg and mg: e.g. Calcium intake = 90 mg/d or Micrograms/Daily.

Vitamins	Daily RDA	Minerals	Daily RDA
Vitamin A	150 μg/d	Boron	20 mg/d
Vitamin B1 (Thiamine)	3 mg/d	Calcium	1,200 mg/d
Vitamin B2 (Riboflavin)	3 mg/d	Chromium	35 ig/d
Vitamin B3 (Niacin)	17 mg/d	Copper	900 μg/d
Vitamin B5 (Pantothenic acid)	8 mg/d	Fluoride	10 mg/d
Vitamin B6 (Pyridoxine)	3 mg/d	Iodine	1,000 ig/d
Vitamin B7 (Biotin)	32 μg/d	Iron	15 mg/d
Vitamin B9 (Folic Acid)	400 μg/d	Magnesium	375 mg/d
Vitamin B12 (Cobalamins)	3 μg/d	Manganese	75 μg/d
Vitamin C (Ascorbic Acid)	90 mg/d	Molybdenum	45 μg/d
Vitamin D3 (Cholecalciferol)	20 μg/d	Nickel	1 mg/d
Vitamin E	14 mg/d	Phosphorus	700 mg/d
Vitamin K2 (Menaquinone)	120 μg/d	Selenium	75 μg/d
		Silicon	ND
KEY: μg — micrograms (mcg)		Sodium	2 g/d
mg — milligrams		Vanadium	1.8 mg/d
/d — per day		Zinc	12 mg/d

Vitamins are any number of organic compounds, each one of which has its own unique chemical composition. Your body needs them to help growth, repair and to run the general metabolism, as well as maintain your health. With the exception of Vitamin K, the body cannot synthesise many vitamins. Vitamin D may be synthesised by the body when your skin is exposed to sunlight, possibly one subconscious reason why humans like to sunbathe. The vitamins D and B12 are not readily available in most plant foods, so those who follow a vegetarian diet would be wise to take a good supplement, but take note that most boxed breakfast cereals or pre-packed meals have these (and other) vitamins added. Look and think before taking daily supplements. Some days you may be getting more than you need and others too little. When taking a daily supplement it is wise to have a combined Vitamin & Mineral supplement which gives you approximately one-third of your daily nutritional requirements. The remainder should of course be obtained by a well-balanced and varied diet. If travelling to other countries for anything other than a week or two it is wise to check up there as to what you need in that country.

VITAMIN VITAL STATISTICS
A more in depth look at what vitamins do for you.

VITAMIN A (Retinol)
It is essential for growth and for the healthy maintenance of skin, the mucus membranes of the eyes, ears, nose and throat, lungs and bladder. It is usually found in animal derived products such as dairy produce and eggs, but carotene, the forerunner of Vitamin A, is used in the manufacture of Retinol; especially in Vegetarian or Vegan products. Carotene may be found in many leafy green vegetables or orange coloured vegetables (carrots). Too much carotene causes the body to store it in the liver and the muscular tissues, in turn causing an orange tint or discolouration of the skin; this may contribute to false diagnostic signs of skin coloration. Too much Vitamin A may also be highly toxic bringing about symptoms of headaches, drowsiness, dry and itchy skin, dry hair, swelling over the bones in the legs and arms, skin peeling, lack of appetite or even vomiting. Vitamin A needs the presence of Vitamin E to be able to store and help preserve it properly in the liver.

VITAMIN B COMPLEX
There are many vitamins in the B complex range but we only need a few in human diets. The B vitamins B4, B7, B9, B10, B14 and B16 were not thought to be essential in the human diet any more, according to some scientists. The fact that Nature provides these though may indicate that they are naturally required. Some of these are now

Vitamins and Their functions; plus basic sources. (Vegetarian/Vegan)

Vitamin:	Function:	Food Sources.
A.	Proper functioning of the cells. Growth of bones and teeth; especially in young children.	Carrots, spinach, water cress, tomato, in egg/butter/cheese and margarine/spread* (*with vitamins added).
B1 - Thiamine	Forms *enzymes* which control the flow of carbohydrates from food.	Dried yeast, peas, Cereal, brown rice, legumes, germ, nuts, some dairy *or with additives.
B2 - Riboflavin	Similar function to B1.	Milk (full cream or skimmed), yeast extract (* as additive).
B6 - Pyridoxine	Conversion of tryptophan into niacin (an amino acid) other biochemical mechanisms.	Vegetables, and whole grain cereals.
B12 - Cyanocob-alamin^	(^) Contains cobalt. Growth in young children and prevention of Pernicious Anaemia if not getting from meals.	Milk, eggs, Swiss cheese, fortified Best as a regular soy milk, cereals, supplement Nutritional yeast. Some Tofu.
C - (L-ascorbic acid)	Skin, healing & viral protection. Note: The consumption of too much vitamin C may *cause* imbalance.	Fresh fruit and vegetables, Green walnuts and rose-hip,
D - Cholecalciferol.	Important for healthy bone growth, Immune System and many other combined functions.	Margarine, egg-yolk, milk + as additives
E - Tocopherol	Employed as an antioxidant. Cell health.	Fatty green leaves, maize, Soya oil, wheat germ, rice.
K - Phylloquinone	Proper blood clotting.	Thick leaf, egg yolk, tomatoes.

re-categorised and I suggest the reader pauses here to research them on-line. For example, "Initially called vitamin B16, or in some sources B15, the product's preferred name is dimethylglycine or **DMG**. Strictly speaking it is not a vitamin, which is defined as being necessary to human body functions, and is more correctly classified as a dietary supplement. Chemically, it is a member of the group of amino acids that includes choline, betaine, sarcosine and glycine. DMG is particularly associated with supporting and boosting the human immune system. This is supported by clinical investigation. It is also used to increase metabolism, to improve physical stamina, detoxify the body and make energy production more efficient." (Healthfully.com)

VITAMIN B1 (Thiamine)
This is also essential for growth, the metabolism and is also partially responsible for the release of energy from glucose. Although it is found in meats, which may not be healthy to eat, it can be found quite readily in whole grain cereals, nuts, pulses, milk, whole grain brown rice, pasta and yeast extract. Any diet that contains adequate amounts of carbohydrates and proteins should also supply enough Thiamine. Vitamin B1 is soluble in water and therefore cannot be stored in any large amounts within the human body. It is also destroyed by heat, especially if in the presence of alkali, therefore we need a steady supply in our daily diet spread fairly evenly in all meals. It is especially important for children as their growth will be hindered if B1 is deficient in their daily diet.

Those who suffer from blood sugar problems, such as diabetes or hypoglycaemia, may have to carefully review their diets and also take a special vitamin supplement that includes B1 (see later section on diets and hypoglycaemia). In adults its shortage may cause fatigue, apathy and loss of appetite. These symptoms may be accompanied by mood swings, poor memory and confusion. All of these symptoms are common, especially in women, when the diet contains sugary foods and *refined carbohydrates* (white sugar, white flour, bleached rice, etcetera) including the 'unseen' culprits in drinks, cakes, biscuits and chocolates (also high in sugars). Stress can heighten the effects and the sufferer may subconsciously desire 'cookies' or other sweet foods as a leveller; this only works for a very short while and the symptoms worsen as sugar levels bounce, even worse again! Women sufferers may also experience worse period problems. The prolonged effects may cause skin problems, eczema, allergies and even muscular deficiencies as the spleen, pancreas and liver are all affected; the blood quality becomes poor and therefore overall health of the organs relating to the blood. See your physician or dietary therapist/specialist or TCM practitioner if you have any of these symptoms. To be diagnosed correctly the practitioner should ask you to annotate your diet and functions over a period of time, if they do not then a correct diagnosis may be hindered.

VITAMIN B2 (Riboflavin)
This is essential to help release the energy from food we have eaten. B2 is found in many foods but some of the better sources include brewer's yeast and yeast extracts, dairy products, eggs and soya beans.

VITAMIN B3 ((Niacin)
Vitamin B3 is also known as niacinamide, nicotinamide or nicotinic acid. It is involved in the metabolic processes and in particular the release of energy within the cells. If the diet contains adequate amounts of B1, B2 and B6 the body should be able to synthesise niacin. Lack of niacin can also hinder a child's growth. Other symptoms may be a roughening of the skin, or reddening of the skin, particularly the face and arms or legs (those parts which are often exposed to sunlight), diarrhoea and other digestive disorders.

Some of the best sources of B3 include brewer's yeast and yeast extracts, nuts and pulses. As mentioned above, B3 (niacin) is one of the vitamins that is usually added to breakfast cereals or other foods, so it is worth checking your food package labels.

VITAMIN B5 (Pantothenic Acid)
B5 is part of 'co-enzyme A', a substance that is involved in several of the metabolic functions. Energy production, one of the most necessary and basic functions of the human body, is included. Dietary deficiency is unlikely with most people. Best sources include strawberries, wheat bran, wheat germ, brewer's yeast, nuts and pulses. It is also present in most oils.

VITAMIN B6 (Pyridoxine)
This is an essential, as it is fundamental in the growth processes and in the production of haemoglobin (used in the production of red corpuscles - red blood cells). It has also been shown to be involved in the process of converting linoleic acid into fatty acids, maintaining the

correct balance of sodium and potassium and the formation of antibodies.

Best sources include brewer's yeast, bread, cereals, bananas, nuts, cheese, eggs and many vegetables. Some books may recommend animal liver as a good source, but when you eat liver you are eating the organ in which there is stored large doses of vitamin A and/or other substances that are harmful to your own health, especially in overdoses!

B7 or Biotin

Biotin, also called vitamin B, is one of the B vitamins. It is involved in a wide range of metabolic processes, both in humans and in other organisms, primarily related to the utilization of fats, carbohydrates, and amino acids.

VITAMIN B12 (Cyanocobalamin)

This is a complex chemical compound that contains the metal cobalt. Vitamin B12 is vital for the proper and healthy formation of red blood cells as well as for general growth. The nervous system needs it for growth and maintenance as it helps to build a fatty sheath around the nerves (like the sheath that protects electrical wires).

We can get B12 from dairy products, especially cheese and also from eggs. Vegetarians and Vegans should definitely look closely at their dietary input of B12 and consider a suitable supplement to avoid pernicious anaemia. Fortified foods such as soy milk (de-fatted) and yeast extracts are a good source as well.

VITAMIN C (Ascorbic Acid)

This is another essential as it is it concerned with growth, including the formation of protein for healthy bones (collagen), teeth, skin, gums, blood capillaries and all connective tissues. This means that it is also an important factor in repairing flesh, muscle, ligament or other tissue wounds as well as broken bones or fractures. Another important function is that it helps the body to absorb iron and at the same time helps the body excrete toxic minerals such as copper, lead and mercury. Even Iron can be toxic if taken in too higher and regular doses, causing IOD (Iron Overload disease); see below. Calcification, a build-up of Calcium that forms in mass, such as Kidney Stones, can be avoided by taking the correct amount of intake daily and drinking lots of water every day, as the liquids help flush excess calcium out of the kidneys and system. Your hair, finger and toe nails are all made from Calcium intake.

Best sources include strawberries, blackcurrant, Brussels sprouts, cabbage, fresh citrus fruits, green peppers, parsley, fresh peas (not tinned), potatoes, spinach and water cress. A diet that is high in fresh fruit and vegetables (seasonal) should provide enough Vitamin C. Cooking will decrease the vitamin content, so raw is better. Raw (cold) foods should be complimented with hot (dry) foods to counter the effect on the spleen, especially where there is a dietary problem such as diabetes or hypoglycaemia (see dietary section below).

Deficiency of ascorbic acid in children can cause symptoms of swelling and tenderness of the joints, sore ribs and difficulty in breathing. A baby may cry when picked up, handled, and if the teeth are coming through then the gums may bleed. Babies are normally born with enough Vitamin C to last them a few months. Those reared on formulated milk should have adequate as it is added. Breast fed babies may obtain enough from its mother's milk. Check with your clinic or GP if you have any doubts.

Adult deficiency may cause sore gums that may become spongy and swollen. They may bleed around the teeth and lead to infection. External skin may become scaly and in advanced stages of deficiency bleeding may occur from the base of the hairs on the legs. Old wounds may break open and healing becomes very slow. This may sound very dramatic and unlikely, but such symptoms could appear after just three months of deficiency!

A common misconception nowadays is that extra doses of Vitamin C will help prevent influenza or colds, but there is no evidence to support this. Excess Vitamin C is passed through the body quite quickly and comes out in the urine. A healthy person with a well balanced diet, regular exercise and good living habits should be far less prone to 'Flu' or colds. Modern working environments such as offices with too high a heat and little ventilation are probably more likely to affect your chances than Vitamin C intake. Try to establish a healthy environment and avoid drastic changes from too hot to too cold. The immune system needs some contact with disease to enable it to keep up its powers; akin to you practising Martial Arts to build up strength of body and speed of reaction in self-defence (emergency) situations. Ginger, honey, lemon and even whisky (a good old 'Hot Toddy') are all effective helpers when you have a cold or influenza. Avoid cold drinks or food as these can exacerbate the condition. Hot drinks and hot foods, perhaps with garlic, ginger or spices will all help.

VITAMIN D (Calciferol)
Also known as **Cholecalciferol**, is a fat-soluble vitamin. It is needed for growth, especially by children and for the prevention of rickets, or Osteomalacia in adults, a bone deformation disease and a healthy Immune System. It should be taken in the prescribed amounts and not overdosed, especially in foodstuffs where it has been induced by such means as irradiation (light induced), or by the consumption of too many foods where it has been added, so risking overdose. Regular overdose could induce such problems as Hypocalcaemia in infants; symptoms are vomiting and loss of appetite, losing weight to the extent of 'wasting away' and constipation.

General opinion used to be that, in adults, the correct amount of Vitamin D is not as important as in growing children. We now know that a daily intake of 20 µg is an essential part of up-keeping the Immune System. This was very much highlighted when several world governments tried to persuade everybody to have vaccine injections against a strain of Corona Virus (Covid-19), whilst ignoring the necessity of Vitamin D. but world experts rose up and, against many odds, promoted the most natural way of fighting any virus, by promoting a healthy Immune System, which is much safer and more permanent than any drugs or vaccines. Of course, fresh air and exercise also plays a part in keeping the system healthy.

Anyone involved in sports, or other injury risk occupations should maintain their daily RDA of essential vitamins and minerals. It is not only essential for growth but also the *renewal* of tissue, absorption of calcium, and the hardening of bones with calcium and phosphorus. More important still is that it helps maintain a healthy nervous system and good blood circulation.

Natural sources include most fish, dairy products, cow's milk, eggs and soya milk. The body synthesises Vitamin D when the skin is exposed to sunlight.

VITAMIN E (Tocopherol)
Absolutely vital for helping to maintain the structure of the cell membranes. It is an antioxidant and is fat soluble. One of its functions is to help protect the food derived substances within the body from the

effects of oxidisation, or 'going off' and becoming rancid before it can be used due to exposure to oxygen. There are four substances that are labelled as Vitamin E and are different from each other but act in a similar manner. These are alpha-tocopherol, beta-tocopherol, delta-tocopherol and gamma-tocopherol. Alpha-tocopherol is the more potent form of these four and is usually the form that is synthesised commercially and used as an additive. It is not common to suffer from lack of Vitamin E, or too much. It should not really be necessary to take supplementary doses if your diet includes a varied fare.
Best sources include avocado pears, fresh asparagus, nuts, vegetable margarine (polyunsaturated, and de-fatted if soya) and vegetable oils.

VITAMIN K (Phylloquinone)
The body needs this for the proper clotting of the blood. It is an essential factor for the production of another substance in the liver called prothrombin; one of the elements that brings about blood clotting after an injury causes bleeding. Deficiency in adults is unlikely, but in babies the symptom would be excessive bleeding. A supplement may be wise but if in doubt consult your clinic, GP or Dietician.

It can be formed in the intestines by natural bacterial action, but we get most of our Vitamin K from leafy green vegetables, alfalfa, broccoli, cereals, egg yolk, tomatoes, sunflower oil, edible seaweed and cauliflower.

SUPPLEMENTS
The vitamin supplements which you buy from health stores or chemists are all different. Apart from the fact that some are singular vitamins and others are varied multi-vitamin combinations, there are also differences in potency and manufacture. Vegetarians and Vegans will want to avoid any form of vitamin supplement (or anything else) in 'capsules' which are made with or from gelatin; made commercially from animal residue such as animal bones, flesh or horns. If you are unsure then ask for expert advice.

MINERALS & THEIR FUNCTIONS
Having dealt with the vitamins and what they do we will now take a very brief look at minerals and their functions within the human body. For a start, all of the metallic or non-metallic elements that are needed by the body must be provided within the daily diet. None can be

synthesised like some vitamins. Their main functions are as building components for bones and teeth (e.g. calcium, phosphorus, magnesium and fluorine), regulating the composition of body fluids (the most important being sodium, chlorine and potassium) and the forming of all other body tissue (this includes iron, copper, phosphorus sulphur and zinc). Without them many enzymes also would not function properly.

Calcium, chloride, magnesium, zinc, phosphorus, potassium, sodium and sulphur are the ones we need most of, over 100 iu (international units) per day. Others are needed in lesser quantities than that. The amounts needed may vary according to age and special needs.

CALCIUM & PHOSPHORUS
They are absorbed with the help of Vitamin D and proteins. The presence of oxalic acid, fats and phytic acid will hinder the absorption of calcium. Combined with phosphorus, calcium makes calcium phosphate compound, which gives the hardness to our bones. The average adult's bones may contain around three pound in weight of calcium phosphate. What may surprise you more is that the calcium is not 'fixed', during your lifetime there is a constant transportation of calcium through the blood stream and it comes and goes as a renewable source.

Dietary sources include hard cheeses, Camembert cheese, cow's milk, water cress, cabbage and turnip.

Fats, as mentioned above, will interfere with the absorption of calcium, in particular animal fats. Phytic Acid, an organic phosphorus compound, may be contributed to the diet within (in order highest quantity first) oatmeal, dried peas or beans, nuts; almond, Brazil and hazel; wholemeal bread and white (treated flour) bread. Calcium is usually added to bread mix to counter this effect. Oxalic acid (highly toxic) is found mainly in spinach and rhubarb.

IRON
Where nutrition is concerned one of the most important minerals is iron. It helps form healthy haemoglobin for the red corpuscles, which transport the oxygen and nutrients around our body. In particular it is the iron pigment within the haemoglobin to which the oxygen attaches on its journey to the muscles prior to 'combustion' and the returning 'spent' CO_2 attaches on the return journey to be expelled via the same

system and the lungs. A wonderful transport system - interdependent, interactive, and self-sufficient. A small amount of the total iron in the system is found in the tissues. Here it forms part of the enzyme system which combusts the 'fuel' with the presence of the oxygen carried in by the blood from the lungs. These protein-iron compounds seem to remain constant, regardless of the dietary intake of iron or even lacking of it. Beware: see Iron Overload Disease – below.

A small percentage of iron will be stored as a compound known as ferritin. This provides emergency rations for short-term deficiency.
Foods rich in iron include water cress, leafy greens, peas, beans, oatmeal, wholemeal flour and bread, spinach, eggs, peanuts (roasted in shells) and prunes. Dried apricots and dried figs are also high, curry powder contains very high amounts, as do any foods mixed or cooked in iron pots.

Tea drinking one hour either side of a meal will both hinder and reduce the absorption of iron. Deficient B complex vitamins may also hinder its absorption, whereas their presence and that of Vitamin C will also help it to absorb better.

Iron Overload Disease (IOD)
American doctors and researchers have found that iron in too great a quantity can act as a toxin and destroy both body organ and brain functions. Iron Overload Disease (IOD) can be detected by the doctor testing for excess iron. Over the counter vitamin C should be avoided as should iron supplements and raw seafood. Natural iron bearing foods should not be excluded from the diet. A natural source of iron is needed.

Symptoms may vary too much to help with diagnosis but can include chronic fatigue, arthritis, heart disease, cirrhosis of the liver, cancer, diabetes, thyroid disease, impotence and sterility. Excess iron can be toxic and can injure every part of the body including the brain. Anaemia can be a symptom. Some anaemia are iron-loading. Iron does cross the blood barrier, it has been found. An excess of iron stored in the brain can trigger or exacerbate severity in Alzheimer's, multiple sclerosis, Parkinson's and other diseases. Psychological problems have even been linked to excess iron It is essential that the patient is tested, following the IOD guidelines, for high iron content.

My old mother lived to a good age, until she was finally killed by MRSA+ due to poor hygiene standards in a NHS Hospital at 94 years of age. At around 87 she started to develop symptoms which were like Parkinson's and was also misdiagnosed by a doctor who did not know of IOD (most do not in the west). Eventually her memory got worse, although she knew me, but though my daughter was her sister (confusion). The reason she suffered with IOD, I could only assume, was the fact that she had two to three bottles of Guinness, every day of her life since she was about 20.

Guinness is renown for it's high Iron content, and in the past has been recommended by English Doctors for Anaemia, due to its high Iron content! There are other types of Anaemia, such as B12 deficiency. There is nothing wrong with drinking Guinness, I hasten to add, as long as you do not overdo it, like my mother did. As they say, "Variety is the spice of life", so vary drinks like you vary meals. If you think you are lacking in Iron, then by all means, a couple of Guinness or similar Stouts will soon sort that out, but not every day! If your Iron content is too high, one of the first signs will be black stools (poo). Stools should be a mid-brown and of regular consistency.

SULPHUR

A non-metallic mineral and component of several enzymes that occurs in some amino acids, which are the elements that maintain healthy hair, nails and flesh. It also helps the expulsion of bile and promotes mental activity. After calcium and phosphorus it is the third most common mineral in the body, therefore quite essential. It is obtained from the consumption of protein foods in the diet and cannot be synthesised by the body. Sulphur is a part of the biotin and thiamine 'B' vitamins and is found in high content in insulin, the substance produced by the pancreas to control blood sugar levels. Sulphur is also found in high levels in the hair.

Our diets in the West are unlikely to lack enough sulphur, but should this happen food of the onion family is high in sulphur content (also Yang food, high in what is generally called Mustard Oil). Nuts, garlic and cheese are also good sources.

ZINC

Although only a trace element (usually too small to measure, but 'traces' may be noted) it is essential for the Immune System, of vital importance for growth, sexual maturation and the processes of healing wounds. Most diets contain sufficient zinc and supplements are easily obtained these days if necessary. Zinc is found naturally in dairy products, eggs, nuts, whole grains, pulses and vegetables, although these may not be easily digested.

IODINE

Only essential for the tissue of the thyroid gland in the human body. It is necessary for the production of the thyroid hormones and is involved in the metabolism. Unlike the other minerals above, iodine may be lacking in our diets. As it is important in the maintenance of a healthy physiological state then upkeep of iodine input must be maintained.

Important sources of iodine are kelp, edible seaweeds, water cress, onions, milk and diary products. Vegans will need to take a supplement. Some natural 'mineral waters' may be higher in iodine that others. In some countries there is less iodine in the soil the further from the sea that one goes. Iodised salt or natural sea salt may provide sufficient iodine; check the contents labels. Do not eat too much salt as the consequence is hardening of the arteries. It is far better to take a supplement if you are unsure.

COBALT

Necessary for the maintenance of healthy blood (see B12).

BORON

In the USA scientific research has suggested that a substance called boron may be necessary for the health of the bones, joints in particular. So far they say that it helps to retain larger amounts of calcium and prevent or relieve the symptoms of arthritis and rheumatism. Study continues.

TRACE ELEMENTS

Other minerals may be found in trace quantities and do not have such great importance. This does not mean that they are not needed though. All elements are important and should be gained from a healthy and well balanced diet. Ginseng root (untreated natural root, sucked slowly, not chewed or swallowed in tablet form) is a good supplement insomuch as it contains many minerals and trace elements.

POTASSIUM & SODIUM

You may recall from the section dealing with the Yin and Yang descriptions of common foods that Salt (Yang) is high in sodium. Bananas, for one example, are (Yin) high in potassium. Potassium and sodium are similar in their chemical conduct within the body, but sodium chloride (salt) remains free within the body fluids. Potassium chloride is retained within the blood corpuscles and body tissues. The kidneys control the action and sodium surplus may be excreted in the perspiration, unlike potassium surplus, which will mainly be discharged through the urine. Westerners are unlikely to suffer a deficiency in their diets, but in some countries like regions of Africa or parts of Asia where large parts of the diet consist of tapioca or sago, deficiencies may be found. The main symptoms would be muscular weakness and apathy, lacking in 'get up and go', as we say.

Remember that the balance of foods is very important and in using the Yin/Yang table one should seek to consume five parts Yin to one part Yang. Eating large quantities of salt (more than a small teaspoon per day) will tip the scales too far in the Yang direction. Bear in mind here that many pre-packed or processed and tinned foods contain high quantities of salt (and sugar). Therefore anyone consuming such things as kippers (smoked and salted herring), corned beef and butter are probably getting far too much sodium via the added salt to these products. Foods with a 'medium' content of sodium include eggs, many vegetables and oatmeal.

Foods which are high naturally in potassium include dried fruits, fish, and vegetables. To a moderate extent bread, rice, milk, eggs and fruit. As you can see, there are many 'crossovers' here.

Vegan Diet.
The Vegan diet is even more restricted than the the Vegetarian, who can at least eat some Dairy Produce, etcetera. What we are seeing now in Supermarkets are pre-produced meals, or Ready Meals for Vegans. Many of these are made with fatty Soya (not 'de-fatted') or processed vegetable extracts and various additives, like Methyl Cellulose, colouring and extracts. These are not natural. However, most Vegans and vegetarians would be wise to take a Vitamin & Mineral supplement. These are not, strictly speaking, *natural* either, but are usually plant or mineral based. Many are "suitable for Vegans", so we have to make simple, informed and logical choices.

TIPS FOR EATING & BETTER HEALTH.

To balance out the sodium and potassium is not as difficult as you may think, all you have to do is eat sensibly: vary your diet from day to day and week to week. More importantly eat (as much as possible) locally grown produce and that which is in season (not 'forced' or grown under artificial greenhouse conditions out of season).

Eat meals that are not too small or too big. Eat three to four meals per day. Chew your food well. Try to relax whilst eating, but sit up straight so the digestive system is not cramped. Sit quietly for ten to fifteen minutes after eating and then go for a walk. If working, try to remain free from cramp and keep as relaxed as possible. If you are in an office environment, eat your dinner out of the office and allow enough time to sit quietly for ten minutes before walking back, also take the stairs instead of the lift.

Concentrate on the positive, not the negative. We eat to live but that should not stop us from being appreciative of the food we eat. Enjoy eating good food that will have a good effect on our body. Many people feel guilty about eating sweets and chocolates, not surprising that these people should then fall ill or be sick. If it is negative and you know it is negative, why do it? Those who advertise their unhealthy products will prey on anyone, even babies (see BABY FOODS section) and children. Many of us are brought up to be addicts of sugar or other bad habit forming things. As adults we come across more information about the harmful effects of these items and are immediately shocked. Shock is followed by embarrassment and guilt. Some people can recognise the problem and decide that with continued will power they will give up the problem food (or drug; nicotine, alcohol, caffeine, etcetera) and change their life for the better. Those that do change their diets and lifestyles rarely look back and feel many times better, more energetic and less prone to illness than those who do not.

Many illnesses are born from a poor diet[1]. TCM has for centuries recognised the fact that many illnesses are related to specific organs or functions within the human body. By treating the symptoms using methods such as Acupressure, herbs and Qigong, then treating the actual problems using corrective diet and exercise (to strengthen the body, organs and functions) we can eradicate many illnesses. This is

---
[1] As far as I can ascertain, it seems that the government and business is responsible for poor diet nowadays insomuch as the cost of living and taxes are so high that almost every family's adults have to go out to work to pay the bills and the high cost of housing. This leaves people with little time to prepare food from basic ingredients.

the object of Ch'ang Ming, to eradicate illnesses or stop them from happening in the first place by altering our diets to be more healthy. This is the ultimate aspiration of all medicine, to be preventative. Curative is only for emergency use and should not be relied upon as a 'quick fix' after we have treated our bodies with contempt. To take this attitude is unfair on health and medical practitioners, for we are burdening them with *our* responsibilities.

We are responsible for our own actions, health and welfare; they are only there to help us in emergencies. We need to educate ourselves into being able to look after ourselves better. There are no excuses, not even 'no time to do anything', as we can all make time or be less lazy or apathetic (another imbalance symptom). Our culture encourages us to eat poorly, become ill and wait until we are ill before doing anything about it. Then we are encouraged to rely on someone else to get us better. This is wrong and a bad way to approach our life. If this description fits you then you need to do something. The knowledge is here, now, and there is no time like the present.

BABY FOODS
The most important time of anyone's life is as a baby. Not just after being born, but even before conception, for this is the time when the mother's body is made ready, or not, for such a precious cargo. The quality of the father's diet can also contribute to his health and the quality of his sperm, a 'living' enzyme that imparts genes and life to the mother's egg. During pregnancy the first cells duplicate and the body begins to grow. Nutrition passed through the system is vital. After several weeks, when the embryo has developed a circulatory system and brain, a life energy form (Spirit) enters the body and awaits the birthing process as another thinking, feeling human being. If we do not eat the right foods we are denying this new life form a healthy start. Most women are highly aware of this and will take every care of the child during developmental stages. Sadly, some do not. Deficiency of nutrition, drug influence of any kind (tobacco, heroin, hemp, cocaine, caffeine, alcohol or even aspirin, etcetera.) can and do influence the growing person's fate of health.

After the baby is born it is fed by its mother's milk. Some babies do not seem to take to this too readily (itself a factor possibly derived from a poor mother's diet or habit during earlier stages) and may have to be fed 'formulated' milk from a bottle. If this is the case, look closely at the labels and make sure that there are no added sweeteners or sugar.

Weaning onto 'solids' takes place from around four months old. This should be done with natural foods, blended finely for digestive ease. No meats are advisable as any infant would not naturally be able to chew meat and digest it naturally. It is wholly unnatural, especially in human infancy. A wide selection of organic vegetables, pulses and grains with stewed fruits are natural and desirable in natural quantities; do not over do something because you believe it to be 'good'. All things in moderation, and like the adult diet, regular doses of varied content. Your post-natal clinic will be able to supply lists of nutritional requirements for infants. If you do not understand something, then ask for an expert to guide you through it. Having said that, not all so-called 'experts' will agree on the meat issue, but take it as common sense, it is not natural and is therefore best omitted.

Baby foods are readily available in the shops, but there is much concern about these. Many contain refined carbohydrates such as white sugar, white flour and bleached rice. These are used as sweeteners or starches to thicken the food into a paste. These are bad for your infant and should be avoided at all costs. There is no guarantee that the foodstuff in the bottle is still valid in nutritional value as shelf life may be long and the contents may be anything up to four years old! Some 'organic' brands offer better nutrition, organic being 'grown without artificial fertilisers or use of pesticides'. However, the same rules as above apply.

The addition of sugar, artificial sweeteners and salt into baby foods may contribute to far more childhood illness than most people would think. One researcher found that a manufactured 'Apple Crumble' contained more sugar than apples! Food labels can be deceptive, for instance; the stated vitamin content may be reasonably accurate at the time of production, but after a while many vitamins will fade off. Food that is left in store or on the shelf for any length of time may not be as beneficial as the label suggests. Deficiency of vitamins, minerals or protein accounts for many weaknesses or imbalances of the internal organs and systems. Avoid giving your infants anything of even a slightly dubious nature and prepare their food yourself. By eating more healthy foods yourself, preferably organic, and using a blender to mix these for your infant you can rest more assured that your child is getting a far better start in life.

HYPERACTIVITY IN CHILDREN

Many toddlers and young children become hyperactive, it is the parent who suffers from this malady. Much of this can be corrected quite simply.

Do not give your child food which contains harmful 'E' Number additives, sweets that are high in chocolate and sugar, anything which contains caramel (including gravy) as well as anything containing aspartame. This should cure many common problems; the aspartame is not connected with hyperactivity but is considered harmful anyway, like all artificial sweeteners, including white (processed) sugar.

Publishers Collins, make a really useful little series of books called 'Collins Gem Guide': 'Natural and Artificial Food Additives'. This pocket sized reference work is worth more than its weight in gold when used to help you eliminate those health destroying elements from your own or your children's diet.

FATS

There is major panic about fats and saturated fats in the world, especially the so-called developed world. It seems that development brings with it confusion, fashions, fads and a whole library load of mental anguish, scare merchants, TV Doctors and heaven knows what else – give me the undeveloped world any day! The question many people ask is, "Should we cut out fat from our diets?" The simple answer is 'No, but cut down'.

Do we need fats?
Yes. The average healthy human needs up to 70g-90g (Guideline Daily Amounts) or 30% of fat in diet every day. That is, out of all the food we eat, only 70g/30% or less should be of fat content, no more than half of that Saturated Fats. Some vitamins are fat soluble, this means that they can not be utilised without fat being present in the body. These vitamins are A, D, E and K. Some of these are essential for growth, especially in young children. Anyone putting a child on an ultra-low fat diet is likely to damage the child's health and growth. Children who are naturally active can burn off their (GDA) fats very efficiently.

Generally, fats provide a concentrated source of energy within the daily diet. Essential fatty acids are linoleic acid (Vitamin F) and a-linolenic acid (Omega-3). These *must* be present in the diet as the body is unable to make them itself. They help reduce Cholesterol, maintain heart health and are important for a baby's growth. These are usually found in plant oils such as sunflower, rapeseed and soya bean oils.

NOTE:
The most harmful fats are what is called Saturated Fats. These are normally found in animal produce and by-produce, including cheese, butter, yoghurt, etcetera. Cholesterol is present in all animal tissues, but absent from plant tissues. The human body makes its own cholesterol, so does not need to import it.

Vegetarians eat far less saturated fats generally, but should avoid high fat dairy produce as much as possible. The odd weekly or monthly consumption is acceptable in most healthy cases, but remember the 30% or 70g-90g maximum rule! Fat intake varies according to health: i.e. obesity, heart disease, etc.

Vegans are even less likely to eat Saturated Fats that come naturally. The word "Natural" is the key. This rules out modern day Spreads, made from Soya, Oil Seed Rape, Sunflower and other substances, but in a highly unnatural way. Always check the label for Saturated Fats and Salt especially.

It is worth noting here that there are said to be Old Taoists, living high up in the Wu Tang (Wudang) Mountains of China who are 130 years or more of age. They are said to survive on Spring Water (not from a plastic bottle!), Herbs from the Forest and an exercise called Ch'i Kung or Qigong (Energy Training, literally translated.)

Diet and exercise go hand in hand. Exercise does not have to be hard, or strenuous. Many millions of Taoists have helped elongate their lives and improve their internal systems, reduce illness and imbalances, all by doing beautiful T'ai Chi Ch'uan and Ch'i Kung on top of a healthy diet. Many western minds are so overly complicated that they cannot understand how such powerful 'medicine' can derive from apparently simple looking exercises. Take my word for it, this route is the best. That would account for why it is *the* most popular from of exercise in the world, bar none!

NUTRITIONAL ADVICE FOR ALL?

When we talk about nutritional needs and daily recommended allowances, we have to do this on an 'average' basis. A detailed personal allowance may be obtained by studying the nutritional facts, the individual lifestyle, current habits and activities. Better still, arrange a visit to a nutritionist/advisor or dietetic practitioner and let them work it out for you based on your personal preferences (e.g.; whether you are a vegetarian, vegan, athlete, steeple jack, land worker or whatever).

If you ask an expert for advice you will get what they have to offer. A nutritionist may offer you advice on the nutritional statistics of all common foods. They may quote meat as being the highest container of Iron (in ferritin form, for it is stored in the flesh - see Vitamins & Minerals), but the same meat may contain growth inducing hormones, animal bacteria (think about CJD for one) and is also high in adrenalin content; as the animals are driven into the slaughter houses they become afraid and the adrenalin which they produce soaks into the meat, you then consume all of these things. Most nutritionists will not be concerned about the *overall* health factors of certain foods, just the nutritional contents and vitamin/mineral balance. A dietician will advise on mainly how you can lose weight or help overcome a certain health problem by eating or avoiding certain foods, etcetera. Of course, not everyone is the same and some may have a more in depth knowledge than others.

Due to job limitations, insurance and legal requirements those who work in the hospital or Western Medical System may be barred from offering anything but 'textbook' advice, therefore some of the subjects, such as symptoms and diagnostics within this book, may not be 'legally' recognised by them (whether they would like to recognise them or not). The simple facts are that, as stated earlier, the Chinese Arts have been around far longer than anything in the Western Medical System, or as they call it 'Orthodox Medicine'; according to the dictionary, orthodox also means, traditional, straight, narrow and unquestioning. The Traditional Chinese Medicine practises have been around far longer and they are not 'orthodox', for we who practice also question and without questions there would be no progress.

It seems a shame that orthodox practises are hampered by a lack of freedom to study and explore, or implement time proven methods. In TCM the main responsibility is laid at the patient's feet, it is he or she that is ultimately responsible for their health, not the doctors or other health care practitioners: they are only called upon to diagnose when the patient cannot and to prescribe a remedial course of action. As stated elsewhere, in the west we are encouraged to let doctors and health care workers take full responsibility for our health. How can this work? It cannot. It is impossible to entrust your health to someone whom you may see once a year, once a month or even once a week. We are responsible for our own health and well being. This book should hopefully go some way to pointing the reader in the right direction.

It is my hope that in the not too distant future, information about foodstuffs and nutritional values, such as can be found in this book, will be taught in schools so that our children can grow strong and healthy and know what they need to do it. Of course, it would also require a major change in the school meal system. As well as this it would be very wise to look not only at the vitamin or calorific content of foodstuffs but also the 'occasional' contents: e.g. In most meats that are not organic you can find elements of growth enhancer (bad for the heart), skin whiteners (mainly in Fowls), plus various drugs and hormones, then there are the extras in fish, such as mercury and other pollutants. These factors can not and should not be ignored.

Since the discovery of many chemicals, so-called scientists have had the brainwave to add these unnatural ingredients to our foodstuffs. You may be surprised to know that this practice has been going on since the 1950's! These additives may be responsible for rises in Cancer or other illnesses, but have in the main not been researched or checked.

Going back to Ch'ang Ming, or Taoist 'Long Life' Diet, is as wise as wise can be. Organic, fresh, local: something you know the history or content of! In my lifetime I have seen quite a few changes top food labelling. It seems that every time something bad is found out about additives or processing, the manufacturers change the labelling or make it less obvious by using a new name or term.

Your life is being affected by modern day scientists who neither understand diet and/or health, or seem to care. They think they are clever and earn lots more money every time they invent and market something. They are remote from the results, so unconcerned. If they were concerned, they would study these issues and change things back to "pure" again.

NUTRITION
THE VALUE OF FOOD

Red, white, black, yellow, brown and pink. We come in all these colours and many more shapes and sizes, but there is one thing that we all have in common as humans, the desire for better health and more vitality.

If you are involved in any kind of sport or athletic endeavour, you train properly under 'experienced' guidance. Your physical health will begin to improve from day one. For a start training will make us physically stronger and more flexible. Physical exercise has an effect on the muscles, heart and lungs, but without nutritional aspects being properly seen to it may be damaging in the long term. If you concentrate on 'muscle work' then your body will eventually get the message and divert oxygen and nutrients away from the internal organs and feed the muscles up. This may leave the internal organs depleted of the vitamins and minerals that they need to work in a sustained and healthy manner. We need to feed all of the body and get the balance right.

If you are one of the many who study the Arts that contain 'yoga type' exercises then you will also be massaging your internal organs into better health and improving the flow of blood, oxygen, bile and waste matter expulsion. With this overall improvement you will feel generally uplifted, of course. Here comes the big BUT. There is a problem with food and dietary matters in the nineties, it started in the eighties and had roots in the seventies and sixties or earlier. Nourishment. In terms of exercise we need variation; stretch, strength, breathing & mind-work. As far as diet goes we need a whole gamut of nutritional substances.

ARE YOU GETTING ENOUGH?
We are talking vitamins, minerals, proteins, enzymes and other benefactors to good health here. The society in which we live is stacked to the roof with things to do and places to go. Even most unemployed people are busy, busy, busy. The biggest problem, especially with the unemployed who do not have enough so-called 'benefit' to benefit them, is NUTRITION. Whole foods or organic foods are not always enough, it is the little things that count. There are quite a few ways that these essential ingredients can be destroyed before we get a chance to derive any nutritional benefits from them as well. Cooking, storage, alcohol and other toxins, etcetera. In fact, if you include drugs (tea, coffee,

alcohol, cigarettes, dope, LSD, amphetamines, heroin, etcetera, etcetera), pollution, contamination, hereditary imbalance, improper lifestyle (e.g; those not in line with Nature) and all the other sources of ill health - it's a wonder that the human race is still here!

Even when the governments are pressurised into making worldwide food manufacturers and processors place detailed ingredients on the labels, there are still problems. A lot of food manufacturers are now using loopholes to group various 'non-desirable' additives under one heading. Although many popular brands of cereal or even tinned foods now contain the most basic vitamins as a 'premixed' additive; these being mainly; niacin, iron, riboflavin, thiamine, folacin (Folic Acid), Vitamin D and B12, it is still not enough to guarantee good health. By eating fresh fruits and vegetables with plenty of rice and other cereals we are also gaining some important fibres and vitamins, minerals and proteins that may not be contained in pre-packaged foodstuffs. What if we pay a visit to the health food store and buy a few supplements? Well, you can spend seventy or eighty pounds to get everything you need and rattle like a pair of Maracas!

Professor Clifford Chee Soo recommended the Chang Ming diet constantly. He could not emphasise enough the importance of giving up all processed and artificial foodstuffs in favour of a well balanced diet of natural produce. This may snag up sometimes on supply and demand; there are so many people who find it difficult to get good quality food in cafés or restaurants and therefore 'give up' their quest for a healthier diet. When you enter perhaps ninety-percent of these places, prepare to meet your doom. What you find in the (very) average restaurants; Red meats, loads of butter, fats, creams, tinned 'things', caffeine and alcohol. In the extremely average and boring café you will find; dead cow sandwiches, processed cheese, bleached flour baps/bread buns and all the other fatty and unhealthy foods. Overall it not only tastes bland but has hardly any nutritional value. It also it might well help you an your way to your first heart attack or even cancer. Even the scrawny alley cat would sensibly walk away from the bins in disgust and go in search of the nearest fish shop!

It is not easy to get high quality foods. Therefore, most people go for a bit of exercise and a few food supplements, such as multi-vitamins. As far as the exercise is concerned, a holistic approach is required. Exercise should include cardiovascular work, muscular work, stretch, tone and relaxation. The Mind also needs to be 'connected' to the body by concentration and control, thus achieving a calming effect as well as self-control.

With the aspect of food supplements, it is a more complicated story. Until recently I was frustrated by the amount of different vitamin and mineral supplements on the general market. Even well known Pyramid Networking Companies offered vitamins and supplements... at a price. Most obviously lacking was a decent product that contained all the vital and essential amino acids and enzymes, as well as vitamins and minerals, all necessary for really good health. If we don't get enough of these we will suffer in the long term.

What are amino acids and enzymes?

AMINO ACIDS: Are a group of 24 organic acids that contain nitrogen. They are the 'building blocks' of proteins. There are 20 amino acids in the human body. Twelve of these are non-essential because they can be synthesised within the body. There are 8 Essential amino acids - these must be obtained through the diet: isoleucine, leucine, lysine, methionine, phenylalanine, threonine, tryptophan and valine. The body uses amino acids to synthesise all the body proteins including enzymes and hormones.

ENZYME: A protein that acts as a catalyst, i.e.; it causes or accelerates a biochemical reaction without being used up in the process. Generally the enzyme names end in '-ase', such as 'lactase' which catalyses the breakdown of milk sugar lactose. They are the principal ingredients of the digestive juices. The enzymes in cereals control the conversion of starch into sugars - essential for sports.

OTHER NUTRIENTS

These are essential for peak condition and performance, maximum health and vitality. Carbohydrates and minerals, as well as nutrients, are needed which will cleanse and detoxify the system. Some people are sensitive or allergic to such things as gluten, wheat, lactose, added sugar or yeast. Watch your diet carefully and monitor your daily input. You do not have to be a fanatic, scribble notes every five seconds or walk around with a pulse metre attached to your body. Just be sensible, give up what is bad for you and start eating more pure foods, more local, seasonally grown and fresher produce. Also eat less fats, chemicals and additives of an unnatural or over-dosed variety. Take a supplement of vitamins if you really must, but do not over do them, one every other day is fine if your diet is fairly reasonable. Just remember that too much is as bad as not enough. Eat small meals regularly and try not to eat meals after 7 p.m./19.00 hours as the digestive system is sluggish after that time and the food will not be processed properly; a sure way to indigestion and fatty deposits.

NUTRITIONAL BUILDING BLOCKS

A successful diet relies on several factors that may vary to some degree according to our own personal lifestyle and intended activities. We all need certain basic substances in order to carry on living, but we may need more of some before we can carry on training, even more if we 'compete' and then some if we are attempting to build our physique up. The most commonly understood of these substances are carbohydrates and proteins. These provide us with the energy to train and are the building blocks for our physical growth. If you train and do not eat correctly then your development will be held back and your health damaged. One of the commonest errors made by young women these days is to train or "workout" whilst dieting. This is sheer ignorance. You need extra food, especially those rich in carbohydrates, to give you the strength and stamina to train, as well as fresh fruit and vegetables. It is after a workout, when resting, that the body builds, heals and will repair. If the right materials are not present then the body will suffer. Powdered eggs, vitamins and sweeteners (aspartame, etcetera) are not natural, so do not expect a natural effect. Let us take a look at these basic elements and discover what we need to keep us active and what they all do.

THE COMPOSITION OF VITAL NUTRIENTS & SOURCES

CARBOHYDRATES: ENERGY.
It is the main source of fuel for all of our activities and takes the form of natural sugars, starches or more complex carbohydrates (e.g.; starch combined with fibre). Complex carbohydrates are the best for us. Try to eat less of the refined carbohydrates; white flour, white sugar or rice.

Main sources; plant foods, wholemeal bread, short grain brown rice, cereals, pulses and root vegetables. There is no carbohydrate in meat, dairy food or eggs and only a little in cow's milk. Potatoes, however, are loaded and are becoming a far too common part of diets.

DIETARY FIBRE: HELPS DIGESTIVE PROCESSES.
Mainly found in what we call whole foods, which are high in fibre. Too much artificial 'roughage' can damage the lower intestines and bowels causing irritation and other symptoms.

FATS: AVOID ANIMAL FATS!
Use vegetable oils (except 'raw' soya), which are high in polyunsaturated fats and have less fatty acids. Animal Fats are normal in animals, not in humans.

MINERALS: GROWTH AND REPAIR.
Essential for tissue growth, repair to damaged areas and for the general maintenance of the body. Calcium and iron are the most commonly known but there is also a need for many 'trace elements' such as, chromium, copper, manganese, selenium and zinc, to name a few. Current research on boron is trying to ascertain whether we need this element. It is thought that it may help retain calcium within the bones and aid better bone health.

Main 'common' mineral sources; Leafy green vegetables, nuts (unsalted), seeds, bread, dried fruits, fresh fruits, pulses, soya products and yeast. A good supplement may be needed by most people to achieve the correct balance.

PROTEINS: ENERGY, GROWTH AND REPAIR.
Proteins are essential for the body. Proteins are 'chains' of amino acids. There are 20 in all and the body can manufacture 12 of these. The other 8 have to be imported via the diet.
Sources: Meat is the highest source, then cheese and eggs, but these are also high in saturated fats, cholesterol and other substances which are unwanted (e.g. meats injected with hormones and tenderisers, it also contains high levels of adrenalin). Meat eaters should beware of 'blue' and 'red' meats in particular. Vegetarians should not overindulge with eggs and cheese. A good, well-balanced dietary supplement may provide all that is needed to level out.

VITAMINS: REGULATE THE VITAL PROCESSES.
They catalyse certain chemical processes within the body (help transform one substance to another) and are essential for the maintenance of good health. We need A, B1, B2, B6, B12, ('B Complex'), C, D & E.

Sources: All major food sources, as listed above. Freshness is best when it comes to fruit and vegetables as the vitamin content diminishes soon after picking. Avoid taking too much of any one vitamin as this can create imbalance or illness. Vitamins A, C & E (ACE) help reduce the cholesterol level of the blood and arteries.

The foods that we eat have to be digestible, that is to say that its composition must be such that it is easily dissolved in the acids that are produced by the digestive system. The foods have to broken-down into minute parts, which then pass through the walls of the digestive system and into the blood stream. Here, salt, for example, is quickly dissolved, meat is not but is broken down by the substance that we call pepsin, an enzyme found in the stomach. (Some researchers have found that the acids produced in the meat-eating processes can interact with the other acids in the stomach and lower-intestines. It is believed that this can be at least part of the cause of stomach ulcers or even cancers.) The results of a study in <u>Cancer Detection Preview 20(3):pp234-44, 1996</u>, stated that in using data gathered from 66 countries, 'death due to breast cancer was most strongly associated with the consumption of large amounts of meat and animal products'. Other research has shown connections with many other diseases, such as osteoporosis. However, we must bear in mind that nearly all diseases are a combination of factors, two or several, including work related, exercise related, diet related and environment.

WATER is an essential factor in the process of breaking down the foods and what they contain. Many of the vitamins are 'water soluble' and can be broken-down easier as long as there is enough liquid intake. Obviously, the purer the water, the better it is for us. Water is also the largest single component of the human body and helps not only to create blood and tissues but general functions of the body, including brain activity.

Most water is recycled in heavy urban or city areas and is treated with aluminium, chlorine and other substances. In some areas there are more natural sources. Where I live, we were very lucky to have our water coming from a natural borehole up until the 1990's when the water authority changed it to a 'standard' supply – not so nice. It was the sweetest, cleanest and most lime-scale free water that I have ever tasted from a tap (fawcet – *USA*) and they had to go and ruin it.

Carbonated spring water is fine in moderation. The body needs some carbon gasses but only in moderation. If you think about it the logic is as plain as the nose on your face, for that is where you breathe out most of the carbon gasses that your blood has just exchanged for fresh air through the lungs! Our bodies try to expel carbon gasses as they are Yin; used and depleted. Drinking too much carbonated mineral water will not do you any good. Also bear in mind that all 'fizzy drinks' are carbonated.

If you drink mineral water whilst out then do not have ice in it. The ice is made from the local tap water. This is a point to be wary of particularly if you are in a hot country where the local water is unsafe to drink; the dreaded 'Egyptian tummy' syndrome! Mineral water by itself or with a slice of lemon in it is very good for you and refreshing. I have noticed that in many places in the UK people in the catering trade tend to shove ice into drinks almost automatically. This often leads to a look of bewilderment or confusion when, for example, I ask for no ice, especially on a hot day. Most people in the west seem to accept such things blindly and I have even seen people in Aerobics classes swigging chilled drinks whilst training – a big 'no'!: sip room temperature water or pure fruit juice, do not gulp.

Two more interesting facts about ice or chilled drinks and foods:
The Chinese, traditionally, did not consume cold food. The reason being that the body has to expend energy to heat the food in the stomach, causing loss of energy, which may lead to pathogens (disease forming situation) or Pathogens. United States researchers are convinced that the consumption of chilled or cold drinks, cold foods or sweets (ice creams, popsicles or lollies, etc.) causes premature ageing in humans.

The most famous source of Taoism and Taoist arts is at the Wu Tang (Wudang) Mountains in China. Here the undiluted Arts are practised and Traditional Chinese Medicine is one. In an article presented by Mr Wang Tao, it is said of hot and cold foods, *"Physiologically, Yin and Yang are kept balanced by eating food which nourishes so that Yin supports Yang evenly. If cold foods or foods cold in nature are taken excessively, they will strengthen Yin and restrict Yang, causing imbalance of Yin and Yang and subsequent disease. In a similar way, excessive intake of hot food or food hot in nature will increase Yang of the body, leading to its over-restraint of Yin and the ensuing imbalance of Yin and Yang, thereby causing diseases."*

Mr Wang then adds, *"For example, excessive intake of raw and cold food and drinks in summer often leads to diarrhoea and abdominal pain, indicating that spleen Yang is impaired by excessive Yin."*

Professor C. Chee Soo used to tell us not to consume cold liquids or foods when there was a Cold present (in the Lungs). The reason being that the stomach is adjacent to the lungs and by placing cold substance into the stomach you exacerbate the cold on the lungs! In my years of teaching and study I have come across many people who have had a cold they "can't move" and have given them this simple advice, plus to have the odd warming foods, those that followed it have made a remarkable recovery from their unmovable cold. Simple really, isn't it.

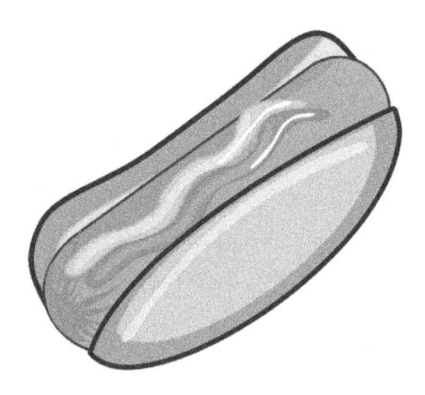

Not so 'hot'!

FOODS WITH ATTITUDE!

Martial Artists, like athletes, firemen, building constructors and many others need energy, lots of it. This should be obtained from the food we eat. Food is anything that nourishes the body and 'Nutrition' is the science of food. There is more to nourishment than just eating virtually anything that is available; we have to achieve and maintain a healthy balance. This may vary according to our output, environment and, of course, the availability of good nourishment. The 'variant' factor can be stabilised by the intake of one of today's multi-vitamin and mineral compounds. The fact is that we need stable amounts of certain substances on a very regular basis. Age, weight, height, sex (female needs vary according to time of month) and energy expenditure rates, plus growth rate and age are all factors which effect and determine the amount that we need.

Speaking as a Martial Art practitioner, we tend not only to work hard but may also become prone to infrequent injuries. With proper and safe instruction these injuries may never happen. It is usually through inadequate instruction or through over-zealousness on the part of the new student that injury may occur. However, if injury does happen, healing can sap your energy levels and may require extra doses of some of the essential vitamins and minerals. In such circumstances replacement is crucial to 'top up' and remain in good health. When you feel 'down' and lack zest for life or training, cannot sleep well or cannot endure physical exertion even for small periods, then something is amiss. It is very likely that in any of these conditions, and more, that you are suffering from a dietary deficiency.

There are many bad habits around when it comes to food and just as many fallacies surrounding our daily fuel, such as, 'a bit of what you fancy does you good'. For a start, this 'bit of what you fancy' may be influenced subliminally by advertising, therefore not what your body is *really* craving for, just your prone mind! Local habits can also drastically affect your diet. If you go to Anywhere-on-Sea, a typical U.K. seaside holiday town, you will find lots of overweight, greasy-skinned people who are sluggish in movement and pallid in complexion. This is quite simply due to the over-consumption of that well-known English meal, 'fish and chips'. Yet another common set of symptoms are observed amongst the people who inhabit other junk-food emporiums and eat copious quantities of beef or ham-burgers and wash it down with even larger quantities of sugary drinks (cola, etcetera). You can see the spots caused by excessive amounts of toxin, sugars and other 'added ingredients'. Fish and chips would not be so bad if it were fresh fish cooked in vegetable oil, chips also cooked in vegetable oil and low in fat. In the past I have had first-hand experience working in a major frozen foods processing factory, so have had close encounters with many alien additives as well as other factors, such as the age and quality of the meat carcass used in burger and other products, and so-on. Additives can be horrifying. In 2005 an American man made a TV programme called 'Super Size Me'. In it he ate nothing but junk food, mainly from the most common sources: e.g. McDonald's, Kentucky, etcetera. His weight gain in a short space of time was quite staggering, as was his reported health loss and feelings of negativity. It took such enormously bad international publicity to force McDonald's, and a few others, to offer a different menu, though what they offer is still mass produced, likely force grown, chemically impregnated, sweetened with added sugar (or aspartame) and probably genetically modified too: as far as I'm concerned the best improvements they could make would do the world a big favour, shut down completely!

The UK permits the addition of 'E 442' - ammonium phosphitides (not permitted in the USA) or 'E 127' enthrosine and 'E 220'- sulphur dioxide. These are widely used and should be avoided by hyperactive children and sufferers from asthma, kidney or liver disorders. It may take time, but some foods and additives are lethal. I call that manslaughter or even mass murder; so why is it legal and why do governments support it?

THE HUMAN MACHINE
To use an analogy, the human body and its fuel system is like the fuel system and mechanics of a car. If you were to put a tenth of the junk into your fuel tank that you put into your stomach, not surprisingly your car would develop bad starting, fouled plugs, clogged fuel lines, burnt-out piston rings and valves, not to mention some very nasty exhaust emissions! So, why do you insist on putting that junk down your throat? And why do you think more of your car than your body? It is not only illogical - you can buy a new car, but not a new body - but also it is detrimental to the environment and other people. By utilising a simple check-list of foods to avoid, foods to eat, essential vitamins and minerals, we can avoid most commons ailments and attain a reasonable state of health and far better overall performance. The most difficult aspect for most people is the beginning. It is not just the will-power, but during the first few weeks of dietary change a 'system

purging' process takes place. All the accumulated poisons, the toxins and other substances are ejected from the body. This gives rise to extra spots by those toxins that are forced out via the skin, plus cold symptoms, wheezes, sneezes, diarrhoea and general debility for anything from a week to six months. And if this happens to you, GOOD! I am so pleased for you as it just means that your body is 'sighing with relief' as it rids the system of the foul. After all, if you were cleaning out your car's system you would expect to flush out carbon deposits, caked-on oils, metallic particles and even expect the odd back-fire! So accept it with ease that you are ridding your system of the dirt and replacing it with new, cleaner and healthier elements that will give you a sportier performance.

Of all the animals on this planet, it seems that only the Human is capable of totally screwing-up its diet and eating all of the wrong things. Conscientious martial artists, and other people involved in athletic endeavours, are one step ahead in as much as wanting to perform to their best. Not everyone is the same though; some are suffering from the effects of a poor diet more than others. With more awareness of foods and diets available nowadays, more people are becoming vegetarian and avoiding the chemicals, adrenalin and added tenderisers and hormones in meat. Many are also wisely avoiding artificial or processed foods, such as 'soft drinks' and sweets, heavily salted or sugared tinned foods, etcetera.

There are a few foods that have a real attitude. They are different from the rest because they have the power to heal or make ill. It all depends on how you balance your diet and in what quantities you eat them.

Please note that the views and opinions expressed in any article herein are not necessarily those of the author or publishers but are included for public interest.

"ASPARTAME - "THE SILENT KILLER"
(An email I received in 1999 from Wendy & Steve in Australia: long since silenced!)

Dear Friends,
We are distributing this article to as many people as possible. It is about Aspartame, marketed as artificial sweetener. If you are concerned about your health, please read it carefully, and take

appropriate action. Please pass this on to as many people as possible.
Regards,
Wendy and Steve.Via / RobNic Group.

WORLD ENVIRONMENTAL CONFERENCE and the MULTIPLE SCLEROSIS FOUNDATION F.D.A. ISSUING FOR COLLUSION WITH MONSANTO.

Article written by Nancy Markle (1120197)

I have spent several days lecturing at the WORLD ENVIRONMENTAL CONFERENCE on 'ASPARTAME' marketed as 'NutraSweet', 'Equal', and 'Spoonful'. In the keynote address by the EPA, they announced that there was an epidemic of multiple sclerosis and systemic lupus, and they did not understand what toxin was causing this to be rampant across the United States. I explained that I was there to lecture on exactly that subject.

When the temperature of Aspartame exceeds 86 degrees F, the wood alcohol in ASPARTAME converts to formaldehyde and then to formic acid, which in turn causes metabolic acidosis. (Formic acid is the poison found in the sting of fire ants). The methanol toxicity mimics multiple sclerosis; thus people were being diagnosed with having multiple sclerosis in error. The multiple sclerosis is not a death sentence, where methanol toxicity is. In the case of systemic lupus, we are finding it has become almost as rampant as multiple sclerosis, especially amongst Diet Coke and Diet Pepsi drinkers. Also, with methanol toxicity, the victims usually drink three to four 12 oz. Cans of them per day, some even more. In the cases of systemic lupus, which is triggered by ASPARTAME, the victim usually does not know that the aspartame is the culprit. The victim continues its use aggravating the lupus to such a degree, that sometimes it becomes life threatening. When we get people off the aspartame, those with systemic lupus usually become asymptomatic (not showing symptoms). Unfortunately, we can not reverse this disease. On the other hand, in the case of those diagnosed with Multiple Sclerosis,(when in reality, the disease is methanol toxicity), most of the symptoms disappear. We have seen cases where their vision has returned and even their hearing has returned. This also applies to cases of tinnitus.

During a lecture I said 'If you are using ASPARTAME (NutraSweet, Equal, Spoonful, etc.) and you suffer from fibromyalgia symptoms, spasms, shooting pains, numbness in your legs, cramps, vertigo, dizziness, headaches, tinnitus, joint pain, depression, anxiety attacks, slurred speech, blurred vision, or memory loss -- you probably have ASPARTAME DISEASE!' People were jumping up during the lecture saying, 'I've got this, is it reversible?' It is rampant. Some of the speakers at my lecture even were suffering from these symptoms. In one lecture attended by the Ambassador of Uganda, he told us that their sugar industry is adding aspartame! He continued by saying that one of the industry leader's sons could no longer walk - due in part by product usage! We have a very serious problem. Even a stranger came up to Dr. Espisto (one of my speakers) and myself and said, 'Could you tell me why so many people seem to be coming down with MS?' During a visit to a hospice, a nurse said that six of her friends, who were heavy Diet Coke addicts, had all been diagnosed with MS. This is beyond coincidence. Here is the problem. There were Congressional Hearings when aspartame was included in 100 different products. Since this initial hearing, there have been two subsequent hearings, but to no avail. Nothing has been done. The drug and chemical lobbies have very deep pockets. Now there are over 5,000 products containing this chemical, and the PATENT HAS EXPIRED!!!!!

At the time of this first hearing, people were going blind. The methanol in the aspartame converts to formaldehyde in the retina of the eye. Formaldehyde is grouped in the same class of drugs as cyanide and arsenic-- DEADLY POISONS!!! Unfortunately, it just takes longer to quietly kill, but it is killing people and causing all kinds of neurological problems. Aspartame changes the brain's chemistry. It is the reason for severe seizures. This drug changes the dopamine level in the brain. Imagine what this drug does to patients suffering from Parkinson's Disease. This drug also causes Birth Defects. There is absolutely no reason to take this product. It is NOT A DIET PRODUCT!!!

The Congressional record said, 'It makes you crave carbohydrates and will make you FAT'. Dr. Roberts stated that when he got patients off aspartame, their average weight loss was 19 pounds per person. The formaldehyde stores in the fat cells, particularly in the hips and thighs. Aspartame is especially deadly for diabetics. All physicians know what wood alcohol will do to a diabetic. We find that physicians believe that they have patients with retinopathy, when in fact, it is caused by the aspartame. The aspartame keeps the blood sugar level out of control, causing many patients to go into a coma. Unfortunately, many have died.

People were telling us at the Conference of the American College of Physicians, that they had relatives that switched from saccharin to an aspartame product and how that relative had eventually gone into a coma. Their physicians could not get the blood sugar levels under control. Thus, the patients suffered acute memory loss and eventually coma and death. Memory loss is due to the fact that aspartic acid and phenylalanine are neurotoxic without the other amino acids found in protein. Thus it goes past the blood brain barrier and deteriorates the neurons of the brain. Dr. Russell Blaylock, neurosurgeon, said, "The ingredients stimulates the neurons of the brain to death, causing brain damage of varying degrees.

Dr. Blaylock has written a book entitled 'EXCITOTOXINS: THE TASTE THAT KILLS' (Health Press; ISBN 1-800-643-2665). Dr. H. J. Roberts, diabetic specialist and world expert on aspartame poisoning, has also written a book entitled 'DEFENSE AGAINST ALZHEIMER'S DISEASE' (ISBN 1-800-814-9800).

Dr. Roberts tells how aspartame poisoning is escalating Alzheimer's Disease, and indeed it is. As the hospice nurse told me, women are being admitted at 30 years of age with Alzheimer's Disease. Dr. Blaylock and Dr. Roberts will be writing a position paper with some case histories and will post it on the Internet. According to the Conference of the American College of Physicians, 'We are talking about a plague of neurological diseases caused by this deadly poison'. Dr. Roberts realised what was happening when aspartame was first marketed. He said 'his diabetic patients presented memory loss, confusion, and severe vision loss'. At the Conference of the American College of Physicians, doctors admitted that they did not know. They had wondered why seizures were rampant (the phenylalanine in aspartame breaks down the seizure threshold and depletes serotonin, which causes manic depression, panic attacks, rage and violence). Just before the Conference, I received a FAX from Norway, asking for a possible antidote for this poison because they are experiencing so many problems in their country.

This 'poison' is now available in 90 PLUS countries worldwide. Fortunately, we had speakers and ambassadors at the Conference from different nations who have pledged their help. We ask that you help too. Print this article out and warn everyone you know. Take anything that contains aspartame back to the store. Take the 'NO ASPARTAME TEST' and send us your case history. I assure you that

MONSANTO, the creator of aspartame, must know how deadly it is. They fund the American Diabetes Association, American Dietetic Association, Congress, and the Conference of the American College of Physicians. How's that for buying immunity?

The New York Times, on November 15, 1996, ran an article on how the American Dietetic Association takes money from the food industry to endorse their products. Therefore, they can not criticise any additives or tell about their link to MONSANTO. How bad is this?

We told a mother who had a child on NutraSweet to get off the product. The child was having grand mal-seizures every day. The mother called her physician, who called the ADA, who told the doctor not to take the child off the NutraSweet. We are still trying to convince the mother that the aspartame is causing the seizures. Every time we get someone off of aspartame, the seizures stop. If the baby dies, you know whose fault it is, and what we are up against. There are 92 documented symptoms of aspartame, from coma to death. The majority of them are all neurological, because the aspartame destroys the nervous system. Aspartame Disease is partially the cause to what is behind some of the mystery of the Dessert Storm health problems. The burning tongue and other problems discussed in over 60 cases can be directly related to the consumption of an aspartame product. Several thousand pallets of diet drinks were shipped to the Dessert Storm troops. (Remember heat can liberate the methanol from the aspartame at 86 degrees F.). Diet drinks sat in the 120 degree F. Arabian sun for weeks at a time on pallets. The service men and women drank them all day long. All of their symptoms are identical to aspartame poisoning.

Dr. Roberts says "consuming aspartame at the time of conception can cause birth defects". The phenylalanine concentrates in the placenta, causing mental retardation, according to Dr Louis Elsas, Paediatrician Professor - Genetics, at Emory University in his testimony before Congress. In the original lab tests, animals developed brain tumours(phenylalanine breaks down into DXP, a brain tumour agent). When Dr. Espisto was lecturing on aspartame, one physician in the audience, a neurosurgeon, said, 'when they remove brain tumours, they have found high levels of aspartame in them'. Stevia, a sweet food, NOT AN ADDITIVE, which helps in the metabolism of sugar, which would be ideal for diabetics, has now been approved as a dietary supplement by the F.D.A. For years, the F.D.A. has outlawed this sweet food because of their loyalty to MONSANTO.

[You can obtain Stevianowin natural foods stores in either cut & sifted dried leaves or in powder form. I use it and it's great.]

If it says 'SUGAR FREE' on the label -- DO NOT EVEN THINK ABOUT IT!!!

Senator Howard Hetzenbaum wrote a bill that would have warned all infants, pregnant mothers and children of the dangers of aspartame. The bill would have also instituted independent studies on the problems existing in the population (seizures, changes in brain chemistry, changes in neurological and behavioural symptoms). It was killed by the powerful drug and chemical lobbies, letting loose the hounds of disease and death on an unsuspecting public. Since the Conference of the American College of Physicians, we hope to have the help of some world leaders.

Again, please help us too.
Spirit of Life Centre, Joondalup, Western Australia. (End of e-mail. Note: Website may be taken down. The address is now only associated with a Naturopathic Healing group.)" (Unquote)

Author's Note: Included 'as is' out of courtesy to my readers and I cannot vouch for the item or any claimed research. However, I have personally witnessed someone who used to take regular quantities of the substance and used to have debilitating pains in her legs, extra weight on the thighs and numbness with frequent symptoms of mild paralysis. It has never been medically proven whether this was caused by the aspartame, but since she has lived *without* aspartame, these symptoms have slowly vanished. My personal viewpoint is that people should be informed of any potential threat, proven or not, and be able to decide for themselves and experiment, if you like, by eliminating substances from their diet for at least a year to see what difference it makes.

SALT (Yen)
This is Mr. Machismo! He is a real Yang monster and will hit you hard if you mess with him, so do not mess with him. Rock salt, the most common, can do far more harm than good. Too much salt (main ingredient being sodium chloride) will harden the arteries, leading to heart trouble. It will also cause the body to retain more water in an

attempt to balance it and dilute it. Obesity sets in. Diuretic foods are needed in combination with a low salt diet to clear some of the sodium and retained fluids.

Other associated problems include high blood pressure, fatigue, ulcers, insomnia and aggressive (Extreme Yang) tendencies.

Sea salt (Tsao Yen) contains many natural minerals from the sea, which are more beneficial to the human body. This must still be taken in moderation though. The Chinese do not put salt directly onto their foods but instead use soya sauce (Chiangyu) or sesame seed salt (Chih-ma Yen) instead. These not only improve the taste of the foods but supply the salt in a way which is much more acceptable and less harsh to the human body. Sesame Salt is delicious, but use sparingly. Do not forget to add up the amount of salt in everything you eat – most foodstuffs bought from shops already have salt added, so there should be no need to put extra on.

IODINE is the only element that we need from salt, but nowadays iodine supplements can be obtained from health food shops or chemists. Doctors will prescribe anyone with thyroid gland deficiency with iodine tablets. Sodium is otherwise available in many foods. Supermarkets are renown for adding too much salt to foods, probably because it 'preserves' and therefore increases shelf life. Every care should be taken to ensure that you are getting enough iodine whilst avoiding over consumption of sodium chloride.

SOYA BEANS (Ta Tou)
This is Miss Goodbody; she is loaded! Ever popular in the Orient, this legume is rich in vitamins and minerals; A,B,C,E, copper iron, magnesium, zinc, calcium, potassium, phosphorus, sulphur and nitrogen, also lecithin which is essential for the health and strength of the nervous system and brain. One useful function is that it assists the breaking down and expulsion of fat in the body and therefore it is of use to those who are trying to lose weight. However, soya has high quantities of fatty acids and these can be as damaging to your health as eating fatty dairy products such as full fat butter or full fat cheeses. It is possible to find in 'de-fatted" form in all good health food stores. Manufacturers are still refusing to label the details and warnings properly. Soya is 'big business', especially in the USA. If you do not see 'de-fatted' or 'de-fatted soya oils' on labels of soya protein chunks

or margarine (spread) tubs than do not buy it. Also try to avoid GM soya.

MEAT (Jou)

Mr & Mrs Party Animal, these guys will pump you full of growth inducers, toxins, adrenalin and chemicals until you are fit to drop. There are more problematic areas to meat consumption than there are advantages. It can supply ready digested iron (ferritin) and proteins in fairly large doses quite quickly, BUT, once you have swallowed it and it ends up in your gut that is where the problems start. It begins to decompose in your intestines and stomach, slowly. An extra 'acid' is created through interaction that scientists claim has a corrosive effect on the gut and causes many digestive problems (obviously these scientists are not the ones who are employed by the Meat Marketing Board!). The toxins may not be passed out of the body efficiently so have to be 'stored' somewhere, so the liver, kidneys and other organs all get affected. The adrenalin, which is produced in quantities by cattle in far larger than the human system can handle, also soaks into their flesh and muscle (meat) and is therefore passed on to the consumer. There are the other problems; artificial growth inducers (believed to be partially responsible for heart conditions), drugs to help fight animal diseases, CJD (from 'Mad Cow" disease), animal blood infections and bacteria and much more.

Thousands of years ago mankind started mimicking the animals by eating meat. In one period Taoists tried eating only meat in their quest for Spiritual Alchemy, believing that the animals were of perhaps higher form and by eating like them it may raise their awareness. It did! They paid very costly prices for their experiments and many died horrid deaths, like cancer, etcetera. This is why Taoists no longer eat animal flesh, especially 'red' or 'blue' meat. Only a very few will eat white meat, like some fish and chicken, but only if it is organic. The flesh of men is the same as that of other animals (muscle, blood vessels, fat and skin), so people who eat meat may be called cannibalistic. Why do those who eat pig sneer at those who eat dog? They are both animals, but everyone knows that pigs will eat anything, even things that dogs would not touch! As Grandmaster Clifford Chee Soo pointed out, "humankind is the only animal which now kills for pleasure. Killing should only be done out of drastic necessity and then only in the direst of circumstances. If man continues to eat meat and become more aggressive then he and she will eventually become lower and lower on the scale of things, eventually becoming lower than the lowest of animals which he hunts/rears and eats!" He suggests that if everyone were to raise their standards of eating, excluding meat, then people may reach the higher levels of their teachers and the wisest sages, thus becoming a an example to all their fellow people. This, he adds, will reduce war, robbery, rape and crime and increase peace, happiness and harmony.

BLUE MEAT
There are still many people in the world who do not know what 'blue meat' is. Shark, mackerel, tuna, swordfish and salmon are fish that eat other fish and can usually contain mercury to toxic levels, especially when consumed often. The mercury poisoning is often found where the fish feed or are bred in the estuary's of rivers which carry pollution from industrial effluence and factory waste seepage. Such is the terrible state of pollution today. It is not only in the air but in the sea and ground.

BRAN
Bran is the fibrous outer husk of cereals, such as wheat. While it is a good source of dietary fibre, especially soluble fibre, it should be consumed with caution as it may cause digestive problems, like Irritable Bowel Syndrome. Most vegetarians get enough fibre from their varied grain, fruit and vegetable diet anyway.

COFFEE & TEA
Caffeine will cause nervous anxiety symptoms and can trigger blood sugar disorders, so it is best avoided. Coffee is the biggest culprit whilst tea caffeine effects are slightly less exaggerated. Avoid if possible. If looking for decaffeinated then ask for 'naturally decaffeinated' coffee or tea as many are decaffeinated using chemicals which are said to be far worse than the effects of caffeine.

GARLIC
Doctor 'G'. The healer among foods, garlic can be added in fresh, frozen, pickled or dried forms to many foods. In stews, soups and as a seasoning its qualities are many; (preventing and aiding healing of?) respiratory problems, infections, injuries, poor blood quality, blood thinner, hypertension, etcetera. In parts of the world where it is used daily as a part of the 'natural' diet, cancer is almost unheard of.

GINSENG ('Jenshen')

The Master. This is the King of all plants. Ginseng can take over 14 years to reach maturity. It is only a small flowering plant with a root about 8 - 10 centimetres long. Tales of its curative powers abound and of course Marco Polo was given some of the finest quality to revive him on his long trip of discovery around China (where it is said he also discovered spectacles being used). It is considered Yang and is beneficial in the countering of toxins or 'toxic headaches', such as alcohol poisoning (hangover!). Ginseng contains many minerals and trace elements that are difficult to obtain through the normal daily diet. The best form of it available commercially is 'Chinese Red Root' which is guaranteed to be at least seven years old and preserved in red clay.

The Ginseng Hunters.

Just as a matter of interest I will tell you the story about the old Ginseng Hunters of China. Ginseng plants grew wild but were very hard to find. During the daylight hours their delicate little flower, which is almost transparent, would be folded up. This made the plant almost impossible to detect. At night the plant would open its petals to the night sky and the petals would shine like a human aura or blue light. The plant is very sensitive and protective, so if any animal or person treads near it, it then folds up its petals very quickly and cannot be seen again!

A clever man thought of a way of harvesting the wild ginseng, which as a powerful healer was worth much money. He employed some of the best archers that he could find. Each had brightly marked arrows and would creep softly out at night time searching for any traces of the radiant little flower, often at the edges of the woods. They could not get within fifty feet, so when they spotted a glowing plant they would fire an arrow in a high arc so that it fell as near the plant as possible and stuck in the ground. Of course, the flower would close up. The 'Ginseng Archers' would continue their search during the night for more plants. In the morning they would come back out in the daylight and search for their arrows, each one looking for his own. Once they spotted the arrows they would have to search the area very carefully to find the plant. They would then dig it up carefully, without damaging the root, and take it to the trader who would wash it and let it dry naturally.

It is said that on one or two occasions a plant has been marked and located at night. Its 'man shaped' root was dug up and seen to have a glowing aura, just like the human body's aura. Nowadays Ginseng is grown commercially on small or large farms. Natural Chinese ginseng of over seven years is the best still. Other countries produce 'force' grown ginseng which is not very mature, tumble dried and then chopped or crushed mechanically to produce powder for various herbal remedies. This is nowhere near as effective as slowly sucking a small piece of 'Chinese Red' every day. With all the pollution in China I doubt that anything worthwhile grows there now.

GRAINS

What we call grains are the seeds from plants that are types of grasses. Wheat, barley, rice, oats, millet, rye and maize all fall into this category. Grain is very good for most people, full of fibre and starch as well as basic essential vitamins, like 'E', for example. Buckwheat is rich in 'E' and you will find that in Eastern countries where buckwheat is the staple food source that illnesses resulting from lack of 'E' are almost unheard of. Vitamin 'E' is excellent for the tissue strength and? kidneys. Barley is good for a high energy level and also for many people who suffer from allergies. Brown rice (short grain is best) is beneficial for your nervous system. Millet (common in the West as budgie food!) is food for the spleen, it is an alkaline and gluten free grain which does not produce mucus in your body; ideal for hypoglycaemia sufferers. Rye is for endurance and helps the muscles and body tissues. Oats are good for those who have thyroid gland problems and like maize it is a good energy food source. Wheat is said to be "a tonic for the brain", beneficial to the liver and high in protein; but also gluten, so to be avoided by those who have to eat a gluten free diet. Rice, buckwheat, millet and maize are gluten free. Wheat and rye are the most acidic.

Grains should not be over cooked and must be chewed thoroughly; chew each mouthful 36 times until a paste. Raw grains can be washed and eaten to get the maximum benefits; try it, it's tastier than you think; we in the West are brought up incorrectly on sweet things, so at first this natural food may seem odd. Eating grain regularly, with fresh vegetables, will provide you with all the energy, vitamins and minerals you need.

MILK

Miss Understood. Quite simply, cow's milk is for cows. Human's milk is for humans. The Chinese mother does not give cow's milk to her baby and may breast feed their child for anything up to five years. Cow's milk is not the best food for mankind for it is deficient in iron, vitamin C and D but contains fats that may not be digestible to infants or very young children. Calcium is its only real value, but that may be gained later from fresh vegetables. There are of course now plenty of alternative baby feeds on the market which have taken into account the special dietary needs of infants whose mothers cannot breast feed any more.

What a pity we live in an age where we are brought up to pour cow's milk on corn flakes and in tea or coffee. In the U.K., where milk is pasteurised, there may be losses of thiamine, vitamin B and C. In some countries preservatives may be added which may also have destructive side effects to health.

PEANUTS/MONKEY NUTS

Also sometimes called Groundnut, they are not really nuts at all but a member of the Legume family. Pulses are an important source of proteins, especially for vegetarians. The seeds of this plant are exceptionally full of minerals as well as proteins.

A serving of just 50 grams of <u>Roasted</u> Peanuts may contain;

Energy	313 k cal.
Protein	14.9 g
Carbohydrates	4.2 g
(of which sugars or starch)	1.7 g
Fats	26.3 g
of which Saturates	4.7 g
Mono-saturates	10.6 g
Polyunsaturates	11.0 g
Fibre	3.6 g
Sodium	0.1 g or less.

This makes the humble peanut a powerful food source and ideal dietary supplement for those who may otherwise lack minerals and proteins.

WARNING: Some people are allergic to nuts or nut oils. Always check with individuals who may suffer from allergies. Likewise, roasted nuts are not recommended for anyone suffering from hypoglycaemia or other pancreas/spleen or liver related illnesses.

RAW PEANUTS: In their natural or 'raw' form they may not be as good for you as they contain some *toxic* lectins and phytic acid. These substances are broken down and therefore reduced by cooking, or roasting.

Vs.

ROASTED PEANUTS: The roasted nuts in their shells are rich in dietary fibre, potassium, calcium, magnesium, molybdenum, manganese, sulphur, Thiamine, niacin, vitamin E, Pantothenic acid and folic acid. In smaller doses can be found iron, vitamin B_6 and Zinc.

RADISH
Mister Radical, this dude is so cool he is cooking. A very potent little root which can help the liver and spleen. Too much is a bad thing and can be harmful. They have a high water content, low sugar and protein. They contain small amounts of copper, iron, folic acid and vitamin C.

ONIONS
Mr. Mustard, he is so hot and will make you cry! Mustard Oil is the hot part of onions, garlic and leeks. Hence they are all good for the colds, influenza, diabetes, asthma and diabetes or hypoglycaemia (blood conditions). They are also said to help those with hardened arteries and poor appetites.

VEGETABLES
Most people associate vegetables with the supply of vitamin 'C'. This is present in most but also other important vitamins and minerals. Minerals are essential for growth, repair and maintaining our physical body on all levels (see Basic Food Properties, above). Vegetables are not just the cultivated variety that most people only see in packs on supermarket shelves: watercress and mustard leaf (salad varieties), dandelion (rich in iron), burdock and alfalfa, parsley, scallions and such all contribute to a healthy and varied diet. To some people some of the above may be 'herbs' and it is true, but this is true of all foods really. All substances which we put into our body have an effect; building, neutral or damaging. Herbal treatment can include dietary reform as all foods have specific values and can therefore be used to counter-balance the effects of other foods; in this context we would use one food to rid the toxins of a previous food, for example.

Vegetables are very easily available and most supermarkets supply a wide range. However, those that we see in supermarkets, greengrocers shops on the corner of our street or even on most market stalls are not necessarily local. For the best results we should take the following advice:

1. Eat those foods that are grown around your locality.
2. Eat those foods that are grown organically.
3. Eat those foods that are in season.
4. Eat those foods that are suitable.
5. Eat all foods as fresh as possible.

POISONOUS VEGETABLES

Some vegetables are best not eaten as they contain certain poisons or toxins that are harmful. Surprisingly these vegetables are the most popular in the West and their popularity is spreading so far and wide that you can even find them on your plate in countries like China now. Mass production, chemicals and modern farming methods have meant that some of these crops are easy to grow, harvest and therefore sell off as a staple; when in fact they are not.

Potatoes (Deadly Nightshade family). High in starch, complex carbohydrates (which are good foodstuff), dietary fibre, small amounts of protein and potassium, thiamine, niacin and B6. Those with a greenish tinge to the skin (thought to be caused by incorrect storage in the dark) contain Solanine, which also appears when older potatoes begin sprouting. These should be avoided at all costs as the toxic Solanine can cause abdominal pain, nausea and vomiting.

In China it was noticed many years ago by Taoist observers, that when pigs were fed regular quantities of potatoes that they became aggressive and intolerant after a while. Many later developed arthritis and gout or died prematurely. So these are best avoided. If you must eat potatoes or are not willing to give them up then do make sure that they are white all through and fresh, not anywhere near to sprouting.

Aubergines, rhubarb, spinach and tomatoes all contain either Solanine or oxalic acid, which can be harmful to the nervous system, reduce brain effectiveness and create apathy as well as other ill effects. Grandmaster Clifford Chee Soo always recommended avoiding these foods altogether.

In the West we may find that trying to avoid such things can be almost impossible. We combine extremely busy lifestyles with travel and this means that we eat out frequently. Restaurants and cafeterias do little, if any, healthy foods: in regards to the balanced Ch'ang Ming approach; not referring to salads, as the average salad contains very little of any use in the greater scale of things.

Even if we eat at home, what happens for the average family? The husband works, the mother works and the kids are either at school, college or university; which invariably means a diet of fizzy colas, chips and burgers, fish and chips, pizza or other fast foods. Mum and Dad come home and prepare the evening meal (often too late in the day to digest properly) which may consist of prepared, tinned or plastic packed articles of force grown foods with "enhanced shelf life" (more chemicals and additives in other words) and, because they have been stored for so long, little vitamin value at all. It is no wonder that the westernised cultures are suffering from more and more illness.

IRON (See 'Iron Overload' in Vitamins and Minerals section)
This section may be of particular interest to those who drink large or regular quantities of 'iron rich' ales, or who consume too many Iron Tablets or Iron Rich Foods.

Author's Note:

Vegetables & Drugs.

Vegetables and plants have been hijacked! In times when villages were self-sufficient, people used to be "hunter gatherers" and men, women and children all had their part to play, meals were variable according to the season. In the Autumn they would gather mushrooms, seeds and berries. Some would be stored, some used right away in their raw state, others cooked to make any Preserves or other storable foodstuffs.
    If illness came around, which it always will, then the wise elder would prepare a special diet, herb or mixture to help cure that disease. Plants like Comfrey would be used for Arthritis or other bone conditions. Honey would be smeared on open wounds to prevent infections, and Yarrow (MilLfoil) used in extremely diluted drops to cure a baby's Yellow Jaundice or liver Disorder.

Nowadays the majority of people have been totally brainwashed into accepting drugs from the Doctor's Surgery for every little cough, wheeze and sneeze. Wait a minute though, most of those drugs are based on plants, like Foxglove for heart disease, so what is going on here? Natural Medicine has been hijacked. The big pharmaceutical companies make Billions every year from dishing out overpriced medicines and the vast majority of people have forgotten how to eat for better health, let alone eat or drink plants that help cure health problems.

It is the author's opinion that we need to stop eating bland diets of supermarket processed foods and get back toward the more natural, in season and local diet. We also need to understand Herbs or other types of natural plants that can be eaten or used to treat health conditions. This is a theme that is subtly recurring within this book. This is also the basis of Ch'ang Ming – the Taoist 'Long Life' diet.
    There are many books written by Herbalists, people who have qualified to use Herbs and know what they are talking about. Why not buy such a book? After you have read, understood and can put this one into practice, to discover a possible next step in your journey to better health.

Diet includes nutrients, proteins, fibre, starch, fats, vitamins and minerals as well as 'trace elements'. Normal diets, even very healthy ones, may not always be able to cope with attacks from virus, or weather related illnesses, so it is then we need a stronger intervention. This is where understanding Diet and herbs come into play. It really is very simple. Tao provides. However, in our built-up, man made landscapes, there may not always be the natural ingredients that you need, so this is when we have to resort to being modern Hunter-Gatherers again and get on-line to find our nearest Herbalist, Herb Farm or Naturopath.

Elderberry.
(Information supplied by Sambucol: www.sambucol.com)

The quite common 'Elder' is a shrub which happens to have excellent medicinal properties. Found in North America and Europe, mainly. Botanical name: Sambucus Nigra.

The elderberry fruit is reddish brown to purple and shiny black in colour. It is therefore also known as black elderberry. Elderberry benefits have been known to mankind since ages, and elderberries have been widely used for medicinal as well as culinary purposes. They are also used as an ingredient in various skin creams and other cosmetics.

In order to derive maximum elderberry benefits, the best thing is to drink fresh juice of the elderberry fruits. Elderberry juice benefits are attributed to its nutrients, which include vitamin A, vitamin B, vitamin C, carotenoids, amino acids, and flavonoids. Elderberry juice is also very rich in certain essential minerals such as potassium, calcium, phosphorus, and several anti-oxidants. If you are wondering how to make elderberry juice, then you can prepare it by extracting the blossoms of elderberry and cooking them. You must refrain from consuming raw elderberry extract.

The health benefits of elderberry juice or the black elderberry extract benefits are as mentioned below:

Elderberry juice has the ability to prevent and treat ailments and disorders of the respiratory system such as common colds and flu, cough, chest congestion, sore throats, bronchitis, and asthma. Regular intake of black elderberry juice protects you against any such ailments. Elderberry for flu treatment was being used by native North Americans as traditional medicine. Since common colds and flu are common and contagious and if someone at home happens to suffer from the flu, you can make use of elderberry for flu prevention.

Since it is very rich in vitamin C, elderberry juice is very beneficial in the treatment of various bacterial diseases. It boosts the immune system of the body, thereby preventing and curing various infections and diseases. In fact, elderberry benefits for kids can be attributed to the fact that it helps strengthen their immunity, thereby preventing diseases.

- Elderberry is also antiviral in action, and as such, it is a potent cure for viral diseases like common colds and fever. In fact, elderberry for colds is one of the most effective remedies to treat the condition. Also, the intake of the extract of elderberry is a useful flu remedy.
- Another great health benefit of black elderberry juice is that it helps in keeping the digestive system healthy. It improves digestion by promoting the secretion of digestive juices, and also prevents ailments of digestive system like constipation.

- Another great health benefit of black elderberry juice is that it helps in keeping the digestive system healthy. It improves digestion by promoting the secretion of digestive juices, and also prevents ailments of digestive system like constipation.
- One of the elderberry uses is its ability to combat cancer. Some of the physiological reactions in the body leave free radicals as the by-products. These free radicals initiate chain reactions that cause cell division, leading to formation of tumours, which later become cancerous. The high content of antioxidants in elderberry helps prevent the formation of cancerous cells, thereby inhibiting the onset of cancer.
- Elderberry is also anti-inflammatory in action and thus can be used for treating and preventing inflammatory conditions such as joint pains and arthritis.
- Elderberry extract also helps prevent water retention (Edema).
- Regular consumption of black elderberry juices neutralizes the harmful effects of bad eating habits and environmental hazards such as pollution.
- Elderberry may help reduce the pace of ageing and makes you look younger. It also reduces the signs of ageing like dark spots, fine lines, and wrinkles. This can be attributed to the high content of antioxidants in elderberry. It enhances skin texture and makes your skin look supple and even younger. It also enhances skin complexion and relieves skin problems like blemishes, acne, and white or blackheads.
- Elderberry juice also helps reduce the cholesterol content of the body, especially the LDL or the bad cholesterol. As such, it helps reduce the susceptibility to cardio-vascular diseases.
- Elderberry juice or elderberry concentrate also shields you against infection of human immuno virus (HIV), thereby preventing AIDS.
- Elderberry juice being a rich source of vitamin A helps enhance vision.
- Elderberry helps treat infections of urinary tract. It also helps prevent kidney and bladder stones.
- Elderberry is a potent sedative and helps induce sleep. It helps relax your nerves and muscles and imparts a feeling of well-being.
- Elderberry extract also helps prevent diabetes by promoting the production of insulin by the pancreas.

Elderberry juice supplies vitamin C to assist in the prevention and treatment of colds. Elderberry juice also acts as a demulcent to soothe the chest. It also acts to induce sweating (a property described as sudorific) which has been commonly held to be beneficial in the early stages of a feverish cold. Elderberry juice also has mild laxative and diuretic (the promotion of water loss) properties.

For variety, try mixing elderberry juice with apple juice, blackberry juice or rhubarb juice. The elderberry tree grows wild throughout Europe and has a long history of medicinal applications. In addition to the berries, the bark, leaves and root of the tree have all been shown to have active properties. The berries themselves must be allowed to ripen fully before picking as the unripe fruit contains poisonous alkaloids and cyanogenic glycosides. The alkaloids are characterized by their bitterness and are chemically related to quinine, caffeine, nicotine and strychnine. The cyanogenic glycosides release poisonous hydrocyanic acid. This compound can be lethal to small animals, but in the doses present in the unripe elderberry, tends only to bring tears to the eyes of adults. While it is important to choose only ripe elderberries, the presence of poisons in the unripe fruit should not put you off this useful berry. Think of the well-loved potato. A green or sprouting potato contains the poison Solanine (another alkaloid) which should be avoided, but this hasn't stopped millions of people from enjoying the standard untainted version.

In bygone days elderberries were illicitly added to red wine and port to enhance their colour. Leading doctors carried out repeated studies to discover that it was only port that had been diluted with elderberry juice that had this anti-neuralgic property. The genuine article had no such value. As a result of their investigation, the physicians of Prague recommended a combination of 30g of elderberry juice and 10g of port wine in the treatment of sciatica and neuralgia.

   As such, intake of elderberry juice on a regular and long-term basis is beneficial for the overall well-being of the body. However, intake of juice of elderberry in pregnancy is not considered very safe. Hence, pregnant and lactating women must refrain from consumption of elderberry juice. Also, there are certain side-effects of intake of elderberry extract. In fact, elderberry benefits and side effects go hand in hand. Fresh elderberry is poisonous, and you must not consume it without cooking. Some of the elderberry side effects are nausea and vomiting. Elderberry allergies are common in most people. Consequently, it is best to seek the advice of your dietician before consuming elderberry juice.

Author's Note:
The above claims for Elderberry are made by Sambucol who create and manufacture a "off-the-shelf" Black Elderberry drink. They claim that the product/s have been scientifically tested and found effective. I have no reason to disbelieve them and have used their Sambucol product myself and found it pleasant.

MAKING CHANGES

So what can we do? We are too busy at work, so cannot cook, and restaurants and canteens are all serving the same old unhealthy foods. You have to think carefully about this, as sudden changes may be as bad for you as the "junk food" or "fast food" that you eat now. Let us consider the essential points of a diet:

1. Vitamins; obtainable from really fresh foods.
2. Minerals; available from a wide range of foodstuffs.
3. Proteins; available from a wide range of foodstuffs.
4. Fibre; available from a wide range of foodstuffs.
5. Water; obtainable from a bottle, tap or spring.

VITAMINS. In order to get your daily dose of vitamins you need to know firstly how much of what you are getting right now. With so much food being processed and prepared for supermarkets there are numerous vitamins (and minerals) being added to almost everything; fruit juices, ready meals, breakfast cereals, instant hot drinks, margarine and other "spreads", biscuits, sweets, snacks, etcetera, etcetera. If you look at most of these products they add the vitamins A, C, E and also D, B6 and B12. Over a period of two or more weeks you need to eat normally but look at the contents panel on the side of any wrappers, tins or packets that you use and then divide the amount of the ingredients amongst how ever many people it is shared by. Write the quantities down for each member of the household who eats their meals from the same source. This will give you an idea of what your normal dietary intake is like when it comes to vitamins. Add to this the average vitamin content of any fresh fruit or vegetables; information available from any good dietary source book.

MINERALS. These are available in different foods and the general rule of thumb is to have as wide a variety as possible. Generally speaking you cannot have too many minerals. In fact there are some which are extremely hard to come by (study the chapter 'Basic Food Properties' above for information on vitamins, minerals and sources). Some minerals, like boron, are so rare in everyday foods that it would be wise to take supplements; supplements are available individually nowadays and not just in "multi-vitamin" packs. Make notes of your daily, weekly and monthly intakes.

PROTEINS. Again available from a wide source. Proteins are the building blocks of the human body, so it pays to know how much of which proteins you are getting. Again the chapter on 'Basic Food Properties' can be your guide. Make notes of your daily, weekly and monthly intakes.

FIBRE. Sometimes called dietary fibre or 'non-starch polysaccharides' (NSP). Less common in most "mushy" foods or not present at all in liquid forms. Fibre is necessary for the healthy breakdown of foods within the gut and also helps to keep the gut working efficiently. Lack of fibre can cause digestive problems, however too much fibre can cause intestinal problems and have other side-effects. As there is no dietary fibre in dairy produce, eggs, fish or meat but plenty in whole grain cereals, fruit and vegetables, vegetarians and vegans are likely to get more than carnivores. Many people eat large doses of fibre added to breakfast cereals (bran, for example) but may not realise that if they eat potatoes, vegetables, pulses, fruit (fresh and dried) and of course wholemeal bread, that they are getting plenty enough already. Some fibre may be added to supermarket products in a form that you may not think has fibre content; cellulose, edible gums and pectin, for example. It is these substances that make up the rigid structure to all plants.

WATER. H_2O comes out of our taps ("fawcet" in USA) and we accept it more or less as is. Its content varies from place to place, from one side of the town to the other, county to county, country to country. We are all familiar with the jokes about contaminated water from middle-eastern countries with hot climates where bacteria thrive in the water supply. Some call it "Montezuma's Revenge!", "Delhi Belly" or Egyptian Tummy. If we are used to a bacteria free zone in our homes and shops, cafeterias and restaurants, then it is no surprise that we are going to suffer when travelling abroad. All the same though, it is just a matter of what you are used to. In the UK there have been many scandals about contaminated water supplies and people suffering. Most folks tend to shrug and say, "Oh well. What can you do?"; which is the wrong attitude entirely as we pay disgustingly high water rates for what seems a very poor service. We have in the UK no government standards or policing which means that even if we buy bottled spring water that the contents may not be guaranteed "safe" to a high enough level, or that it does not contain in that batch higher phosphates or whatever else is washed through the farmland into the underground springs. Many people may suffer from pollution or poisoning; take the aluminium used by one South-West company which was tipped into the wrong tank causing local grief and untold suffering; and they still have not been big enough to stand up and admit their guilt and responsibility fully.

So when it comes to water, well (no pun intended) I prefer mountain spring or boiled for tea. We need liquids. Just be wary about how you get them; sugary drinks, and caffeinated coffee may quench your thirst but what else are they doing?

By taking the course of action outlined in the above five categories you can build up a picture of your daily, weekly and monthly intakes. From this consciousness you will have the choices of what you will choose to do about it. Vitamin and mineral substitutes (supplements) are not always the best way of getting the right things but sometimes they may be the only way. It is not my place to say that you should or should not have this or that, for I am here to act purely as a guide and to enlighten you. It is your place and your own conscience by which you must make the daily decisions by which you live or die.

Foods with attitude are quite amazing, for they can kill or cure, but one thing is for certain, poison is poison. All that I can relate to you are my personal experiences. It is a fact that I feel better at fifty than I did at fifteen, I have more level energy, less illness and better stamina. My sleep is brilliant and my body is firm and strong. The only time I get headaches is when I have spent too many hours at the computer (writing these books and articles) and have assumed an uncomfortable working position, or when I have had the wrong kind of beer (I discovered that Wheat Beer does not like me at all!). Apart from the odd "wobble" I feel truly great. This is due to my participation in Quanshu ('Kung-fu', to use the slang) and T'ai Chi Ch'uan (Taiji Quan), Ch'i Kung (Qigong) and of course a healthier vegetarian Ch'ang Ming Diet; not perfect yet but I am getting there, listing and loosing.

My advice is simple; avoid one item that we know is bad for you from your diet. Replace it with a healthy option chosen from this book's lists and information. Once you have adapted to that you can later look at another optional food and replace that. Slowly but very surely you will notice changes in yourself, less headaches, less influenza, colds or other common ailments.

As an example, a smoker could cut down on her or his intake (please be aware of those around you as 90 percent of the smoke goes into the atmosphere and is known to contain 160 cancer causing chemical agents!). Be aware of the facts that the tar will block the delicate lining of the lungs through which the air you breathe should pass into the bloodstream; the tar and nicotine then filters into the blood, causing arterial restrictions leading to heart attacks. Cancer in other organs is caused by these circulation problems and generally the brain is affected adversely. The stomach is also affected and cancer again is one of the most common outcomes around the gut area. So called "passive smokers" who are forced to breathe in the polluted air can suffer cancer, asthma or common colds and flu (influenza) symptoms due to the effects of smoke inhalation.

There are many other drugs to get hooked on, such as chocolate (I see anything of an addictive nature, taken for "comfort" as a drug, for the effects and causes are similar and the addiction starts off as mental weakness followed by physical induction and supposed mental need (caused by chemical changes)). There is no real need for these substances, counselling is what is really needed, even if only to talk it out with a good friend.
The old excuse is, "Yeah! It's easy for you to say." So what makes you think that? I've had to change things in my life and if I can do it so can you. There are some minor things that I still need to work on. Like every great journey, it begins with one step forwards. "Yeah, but my need is greater than yours.... My problems you wouldn't understand." is the usual follow on. Nobody has problems any greater than the next person; they are merely of a different structure, but still only questions that need to be understood. It is this you have to work on; understand the situation and the problem no longer exists. It is like a puzzle; it is only a puzzle until you have solved it and then it all becomes amazingly clear and simple.

Our lives are filled with temptations to eat, drink, smoke or even inject all sorts of things into our already overworked bodies. Advertisers, drug pushers (legal and illegal), sweet makers and sellers all want us to buy their products on the premise that they will make us feel better.

Bombarded by this constant sales pitch we succumb and do it. The result is that we then get lost in that "forbidden fruit" (as the advertisers put it so often) and immerse ourselves into a chemically altered state whereby we tend to forget, for the moment, all of our problems. In reality we are adding another problem. Putting another layer of dirt on the window of our consciousness.

LIST AND LOSE

In a way, this is the most important section of the book. This is the test, the wake up call, and the point that could change your life. The way out is to work on our personal consciousness and to do this we must say, "Stop!" Take a look at what we are doing to ourselves and then reaffirm that we are going to make changes, albeit small ones at first. Make a list of all the things which are being consumed as "comfort" items (this can even include shopping sprees) and then take items from that list which you think are number one to lose, second to lose, third to lose and so on. Underline number one and tell yourself that from today you will not do, take, indulge or whatever with that item for just one short week; you will not miss it as there are plenty of normal chores and things to keep you occupied. After a week you must sit down and honestly evaluate your week of abstention. You will find that you did not miss this food, drug or whatever your particular addiction was. The facts are that if you can avoid it for a day, a week means that you can live without it forever!

BEING POSITIVE

The next step is to affirm that the loss is good, "I'm right. I don't need it at all. In fact I'm much happier and healthier without it. I feel great!" Repeat this affirmation several times. During the second week look at your list and start planning a week without the second item. At this stage we need to replace the item with something worthwhile, like a discovery walk of the local area, or visit a friend (you can tell them how good you have been), or just go "chill out" and relax in the park with a good book. After the second week of abstinence from item one, item two can be worked on and the affirmations become more natural, "I really didn't need that at all. I'm feeling so much better without them. I'm doing really well and feeling much better and more positive!" At this stage it might be a good idea to plan a holiday or use some of the money you have saved improving your living environment; decorate or a new sofa, hi-fi or whatever. Before you know it you will be working your way through the list and making new plans, giving up more "junk", drugs and other things that make your windows dirty in favour of more natural things; and how good it feels.

A Final Case History:
Myself.

In 1970 I decided to become vegetarian. It was for health as well as moral reasons as red meat was giving me really bad migraines and other problems. My Father also died prematurely, partially due to excess meat eating, partially salt and smoking too. Not long after he died, I took this as a hint to myself that I should learn more about food and diet. That I did. When I first quit eating animal flesh, it was hard. For the first six months or so I had spots, wheezes, coughs and sneezes, but this was just my body breathing a sigh of relief as it kicked out the toxic waste which accumulates after years of poor dietary intake. My taste buds slowly became better and I enjoyed my food more. The simple things became so much better, even plain wholemeal bread tasted so good compared to its stodgy and 'rubbery' white cousin.

After reading George Oshawa's book on Zen Macrobiotics I decided that I would take a bigger step. In the early summer of 1971 I went on the purging and cleansing Brown Rice Diet. This consisted of fasting for at least one to two days; just a sip of water if you are thirsty. The following days I increased my water intake and ate only washed, short grain brown rice (uncooked) by chewing each portion at least thirty-six times or until it all became a fine paste. My body rid itself of many more toxins and felt different. Even though I had eaten less I felt stronger, my sleep was better, my energy on waking was bright and even and my days were far more enjoyable.

After a fortnight I had built up to "normal" meals and had a natural breakfast, lunch and evening meal, but the foods were more pure and I had given up meat and other items. As an addition I sucked some 'Chinese Red' Ginseng root each day in the ancient prescribed manner. Three times each day I would walk from where I lived in Caister-on-Sea to Great Yarmouth to see my friends. On the way I would gather or spread seeds from trees and shrubs to help preserve wooded areas that we need for our oxygen and cleaner air. My awareness became incredible and often my attention would be alerted to a cat or a bird looking at me from behind or above. My 'Kung-fu' became better and my training took on a new lease of life. Above all I was more at peace with myself and even though life is still a struggle sometimes, the power is there. This lead me to giving up many more things which were harmful to me and now, as then, I never, ever give up or go backwards! To this day (51 years to 2021) my life feels better and I feel more fit and strong all the time. It is owed to the Oriental Arts and the wisdom of (mainly) the ancient Chinese.

SUMMARY

There you have it, foods with attitude and attitudes with food. If you follow the steps in the 'List and Lose' section you will be able to make changes that dramatically affect your life. These changes may be dramatic, but they are not ones which will make you frightened, just amazed at how much better you can feel. Awareness is the key. To become aware of what ails us we must be aware of what we consume, the environments in which we work, shop and live (fumes, sprays, materials, etcetera) as well as the contents of our food and drink. Start reading labels, looking at reference books and learning about *your* life. You will become aware of many things that are harmful to your health and many which are beneficial and more enjoyable as a result (another Yin & Yang effect!). Above all, remember that old Chinese proverb which applies to so many things in our life; "Every great journey of a thousand miles begins with just one step."

Personal Enquiry

Do you think that being a vegetarian means that you will be weak? Do you think that meat gives you strength and stamina? If you do, then why do you think these things? In all likelihood your perceptions will be based upon what you were told by your parents, and them by their parents. These perceptions are often founded on hearsay, "old wives' tales", advertising and reports generated by parties who have invested interests: e.g. The Meat Marketing Board, who may pay a food scientist to publish a report finding something positive about meat, but omitting all the negative points. Such is life.

Think about the above honestly before reading on.

Contemplation

Should you be one of the many generations who was brought up with old wives tales and superstitions, but nothing much based upon fact, and if you were raised to believe that you need meat to be strong, the following facts may be rather surprising to you.

Some very interesting and noteworthy vegetarians/vegans include, Carl Lewis (Nine times Olympic Champion Sprinter), Martina Navaratilova (Nine times Wimbledon Tennis Champion), Robert Miller (British Cycling Champion), Steven Seagal (Martial Arts performer/actor), Edwin C. Moses (Olympic Champion Sprinter and Hurdler), Chris Campbell (World Champion Wrestler), Murray Rose (Australia: Four times Olympic Gold Medallist Swimmer), Ms Elena Walendzik (German Featherweight Boxing Champion 2005), Luiz Freitas (Brazilian Body Builder Champion), and let us not forget the beauty and the brains of Christy Turlington (Supermodel), Bob Dylan, Henry Ford, Kate Winslet, Ashley Judd, Demi Moore, Joan Baez, Charles Darwin, Socrates, Leonardo Da Vinci, Pythagoras (mathematician/philosopher), Albert Einstein, Richard Gere, Jesus Christ (who, according to a BBC Documentary, might have been a Buddhist, or at least spent much time learning about health and healing at Buddhist retreats), The Dali Lama of Tibet, and of course the beloved 'Patron father' of Taoism, Lao Tzu (left). To name just a few!

More recently, a Vegan woman named **Yolanda Presswood (pictured below)** made history when she broke the Californian and US Power Lifting record for Squat, with just *one* repetition, and the state record for Bench. This earned her the title of Best Masters Lifter as well as first place. According to Great Vegan Athletes the athlete's Squat saw her lift an impressive 128 kg (283 lb) and Bench Press 62.5 kg (137 lb). That's incredible going. Other modern day celebrities who are Vegan, include Lewis Hamilton (Formula 1), boxer David Haye, Tennis power-house Serena Williams, Jehina Malik - Body Builder, Boxer Mike Tyson, Snowboarder Hannah Teter and Cyclist David Zabriskie.

All researched on-line, I am sure you can find more.

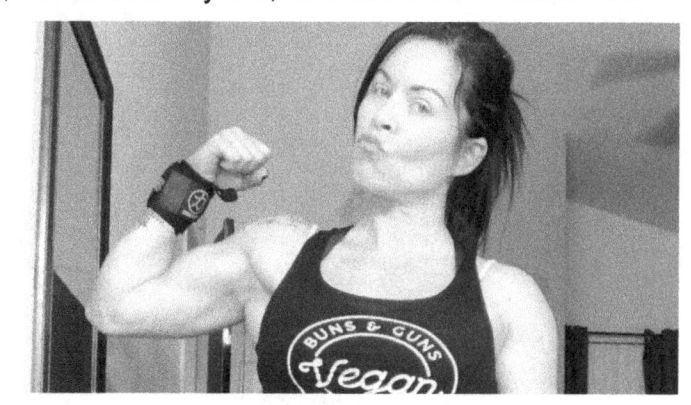

SPECIAL NEEDS SECTION

ARTHRITIS - 165

CANCER – 173

HYPOGLYCAEMIA - 183
& Hyperglycaemia - 190

IRRITABLE BOWEL SYNDROME – 193

VIRUS – Eat to Beat Covid - 199

Some very common ailments that can be avoided or helped by changing to and sticking with a better, healthier diet.

ARTHRITIS
OSTEOARTHRITIS
RHEUMATOID ARTHRITIS

ARTHRITIS

One of the most common diseases around, inflammation of the joints affects millions of people, young as well as mature. It causes problems with the finger joints, shoulders and neck and can bring great discomfort as well as pain. Research is still going on into the causal effects of arthritis, but whilst elemental and environmental factors (because of their complexity) still elude the scientists we have been able to pinpoint certain problems with the dietary aspects.

Rheumatism is a term generally referring to any pains around the joints or muscles in the limbs or body. Arthritis refers to damage of the joints, although 'rheumatoid disease' is often used as an umbrella term for any form. There are thought to be around 200 forms of rheumatic disease by orthodox practitioners (your general practitioner and local hospitals are orthodox). They categorise them into four groups for better recognition.

1) Inflammatory Arthritis; the joint becomes inflamed and the surface lining of the joints and underlying bones can become damaged; Rheumatoid arthritis is usually grouped here. Gout, reactive arthritis, arthritis connected with psoriasis or colitis and other disorders of the joints or bones which may not be "fully understood" as yet by Western Medicine.

2) Osteoarthritis; a common disorder where the surface of the joints becomes damaged and worn, or pitted as though eaten away and abnormal stress is then placed upon the joints. The hips, knees and hands are most commonly affected.

3) Rheumatism of the (soft) tissues; Western Medicine sees this as short term arthritis caused by injuries to the ligaments and tendons around joints, perhaps through sport or work related causes. Fibrositis and fibromyalgia are lumped into this category.

4) Back Pain; Orthodox practitioners tend to think of this mainly as problems related to the muscles, spinal column discs and ligaments around the back area.

Generally, orthodox medicine thinks of arthritic diseases as a problem that "develops", presumably for no reason, and then affects the body in various ways. Traditional Chinese Medicine thinks upon it as a condition which is brought about by an imbalance, injury or lacking in the bodily functions. Although severe cases (osteoarthritis) may be too advanced to cure, dietary changes can effect some relief. Carefully monitoring our diets from an early age may help prevent arthritic disease from forming at a later date. Again this 'prevention rather than cure' philosophy prevails in TCM.

A big concern is children's diets. There is concern in schools that poor diets and foods high in sugar and processed elements cause bad behaviour, hyper-activity and diminishing attention span. Many parents are pushed for time so tend to go for the quick and easy option without reading labels or thinking about the content. Teenagers like to think that they are fending for themselves and buy 'junk food' from the proliferation of junk food emporiums.

Some people suspect that arthritis may be passed on in family genes. This may be true insomuch as susceptibility is passed on. It is more likely that if anything is passed on, it would be through dietary faults (traditional family meals) and local country or area soil mineral deficiencies, etcetera. Orthodox medical scientists are also looking at the possibility of environmental factors; pollution, infections, climatic conditions. Who knows, they may come up with something of interest here.

COMMON SYMPTOMS

SWOLLEN JOINTS • STIFFNESS IN OR AROUND JOINTS • PAINFUL TO MOVE JOINTS • TIREDNESS • GENERAL DEBILITY OR UNWELL FEELING • PERSISTENT PAINS AROUND JOINTS • STIFF OR ACHING BACK AND/OR LIMBS, NOT DUE TO EXERCISES • WEIGHT LOSS • NIGHT SWEATS • MILD FEVER • SKIN RASHES •

FIVE ELEMENT THEORY
In TCM, the Chinese Health Practitioners believe that all of these conditions relate directly to the state of nourishment within the human

body; food, liquids and Qi. In the Wu Hsing Theory (see the section above dealing with the Five Element Theory and how each element relates to the other) these diseases relate to the Greater Yin/Water and Kidneys. The bones and nails being affected here by cold, frost and icy conditions. Changes in climatic conditions may aggravate and therefore heighten pain or reduce it. The correct foods will however replenish those vitamins and minerals the body lacks and stay off the effects; depending on the severity of the condition.

In the Wu Hsing cycle this strain on the kidney functions could have been caused by the liver "drawing from it" whilst it dysfunctional. The liver controls the muscles and tissues. Wind will aggravate as will dry or crisp conditions. So by treating the liver condition we can hope to strengthen the cycle and by treating the depleted kidneys repair the damaged cycle and regain a balance.

The kidneys, as seen in the Five Element Table, are in control of the bones; where arthritic disease is felt. Winter is the worst time and frost or ice should be avoided. Night time may feel worse and cold conditions will aggravate. Thermogenisis is the treatment recommended but dietary reform is a must. One of the biggest problems with the human race is there ability to take good, wholesome foods, leave them aside and invent a new diet which comprises of nothing more than artificial proteins, chemicals and processed sugars, etcetera. "Rubbish", that which pollutes our bodies and causes ever more common ailments amongst us. If we do not stop this dietary and polluting madness now by the year 2500 we will see an increasing amount of babies born with new health problems, deformities and defects. We must learn to eat naturally the Ch'ang Ming way.

WESTERN MEDICINE: It is now known that 'free radicals' (destructive oxygen molecules) cause damage to the cartilage of the joints, especially in the over 70's, which helps bring about osteoarthritis. This condition, nutritional experts believe, is brought about by high levels of tissue acidity and "pollution" of the body, plus a lack of anti oxidising vitamins and minerals.

TCM: This situation is known to the Chinese. When too many toxins are taken in, the kidneys are "overloaded" and cannot eradicate the excessive amounts from the system. This excess then has an accumulative effect and will permeate elsewhere, polluting the kidneys and then the rest of the system. Western medical science is slow, but they are at least on the way to understanding what the Traditional Chinese Medicine practitioners have known for centuries!

FOOD FACTORS.

Amazingly, Western Orthodox Medicine has begun to realise the connections; though arguments still persist as some medical scientists appear to value personal fame and fortune in their quest to make pharmaceutical history by inventing yet another drug to sell by the millions to the "guinea pig" masses. Experimentation goes on in all fields of medicine with human subjects. Many people have been told by their family doctors that the pills they are given are "new" so they ask that all side-effects or feelings are reported. This information goes back to the drug manufacturers who then may experiment further or scrap it for the next "super drug" and try again. In sheer desperation, and because drugs do not rid arthritic conditions, they are turning to diet. Hooray! In 1970 my Taoist Arts Master, Grandmaster C. Chee Soo, helped many people with bone, joint and muscle conditions (see main book sections) to overcome their pains and disability. How? With simple dietary reform and gentle exercise; the Chinese are far, far ahead of Western Medicine and always have been.

FOODS TO BE AVOIDED:

Red Meats; beef, lamb, pork/ham.
Dairy Foods; cow's milk, yoghurt, cheese (especially full fat).
Coffee, tea, cocoa and *alcohol.
Sugars; (white 'beet' sugars), also syrups and treacle.
Nuts; especially peanuts and dry roasted nuts.
Fruit; blackcurrant, grapefruit, gooseberries, lemons, limes, oranges, strawberries.
Vegetables; potatoes (solanine of the Nightshade family), aubergine (Eggplant), tobacco, peppers, rhubarb. Vegetable Cooking Oils for Frying.
Flour; brown and white.
Sundries; salt, pepper, pickles, vinegar.

Closer Detail.
Alcohol: It is formed by fermenting sugar. Alcohol, also known as ethanol or ethyl alcohol, is readily absorbed through the stomach and intestines into the blood stream. When it reaches the liver it is converted

into Acetaldehyde. The consumption of alcohol suppresses the enzyme Delta-6-desaturase, an enzyme that helps convert essential fatty acids into Gamma-linolenic-acid (GLA) and Eicosapentaenoic-acid (EPA). According to Linda Lazarides' in her excellent book, treatment of heavy drinkers with supplements of GLA and EPA have proven quite successful against arthritis.

She adds, "Alcohol also interferes with the metabolism of folic acid and methionine. The risk of breast cancer increases in women who consume three or more drinks a day".

Since alcohol also interferes with and depletes anti oxidants Vitamin B, these elements being necessary to mitigate the free radicals, it makes sense to cut out or cut down. Many people, including my dear old mother, like to have an Irish Stout drink, rich in iron and proteins. This is usually seen as "acceptable", but in moderation as three or more a day will be too many. It must also be remembered that "shorts" (whisky, vodka, rum, etcetera), although being such a small drink, are high in alcohol levels.

SUPPORTIVE FOODS.

Pulses: Beans, lentils and peas (legumes), plus linseed, sunflower* and pumpkin seeds.
Dairy: Goats' milk and cheese, soya milk or cheese (de-fatted). Halloumi is good in moderation but is high in Salt & Saturated Fats.
Meat: not advised generally but cod or haddock (white fish, deep sea).
Nuts: Almond, cashew, pecan and walnuts.
Vegetables: Broccoli, cabbage, celery, beetroot, leafy greens, lettuce, marrow, parsley, seaweed (Kombu, Wakame, etcetera.), swedes, turnips, watercress.
Grains: Buckwheat, barley, millet, rice (brown, short grain).
Fruits: Grapes, melons, sun dried (figs, prunes, raisins & sultanas), other fruits now widely available.
Oils: *Sunflower oil, "pure" and margarine (avoid impure brands).
Drinks: Herbal teas, spring water, dandelion coffee, unsweetened fruit juices (but *not* acidic "citrus" fruits, including orange), vegetable juices and or vegetable stocks.
Flour: Corn cakes/flour, oats/oat cakes, millet, rice flour, rye and rye crisp breads, tofu.
(Warning: *Always read food content labels!*)

*Detail: Many people take supplements for oils, such as "cod liver oil", an extract from the codfish's liver. This is usually high in Vitamin A, E and other substances, some of which may be toxins stored by the liver. Excess of these vitamins and minerals can be extremely harmful and even fatal. Use sunflower oils on salads, pasta or even in soups, just a spoonful a day will help your arthritic problems.

Vitamin & Mineral Supplements.

Vitamins: C, B complex, D and E.
Minerals: Calcium, copper, iron, magnesium, molybdenum, selenium and zinc.

Amino Acids: Cysteine, glutathione, methionine and phenylalanine.
Sundry: Borage oil, Evening Primrose oil.

Exercise: The body always needs exercise to increase circulation and enhance the digestion of food; a gentle walk 15 minutes after eating, for example. Exercise will help stimulate the other processes in the body and that includes the transformation and circulation of proteins and nutrients. On a more general note exercise will keep the muscles, ligaments and other tissues healthier. Many rheumatic and arthritic sufferers have found great relief from doing T'ai Chi Ch'uan (Taiji Quan) exercises every day, early morning and before bed. In China a doctor may send you along to join a Taiji class as well as recommend a better diet!

You can find classes or groups in your area by looking at notice boards in your local community centers or asking for information at local libraries. Sometimes classes are advertised in the press or 'free-ads' papers. A Chinese man now living and working in Australia as a general physician, Dr Paul Lam, suffered from arthritis in his youth. His doctor told him to take up T'ai Chi Ch'uan/Taijiquan: sometimes written as "Tai Chi". This he did and became so good he even won a gold medal at the Peking Games. Apart from that he noticed a tremendous relief from the symptoms of arthritis. Working with some of the top arthritis specialists in Australia he has developed a set of warm up exercises and a short T'ai Chi Form, based on Sun Style, that is especially good for arthritis sufferers.

You can find information about Tai Chi for Arthritis from this website about classes and instructors Internationally: www.taichiproductions.com

Since this book was first published, in the 1980's, the Internet has flourished and the WWW is truly world-wide, to the extent where people can view and access it on Mobile Phones. There are now many websites promoting T'ai Chi Ch'uan/Taijiquan, Qigong and other related and beneficial Arts. Finding a teacher may be easier now than ever, but you still need to find a good one! You are always best to look around, ask questions and, best of all, ask students what classes or instructors are like.

There are other forms of exercise that are good for arthritis sufferers. There is a 'new safer standardised' set of Baduanjin – The Eight Strands of Silk Brocade. This is a truly delightful set of eight simple qigong exercises which can be done standing, there is also a seated set, and without strain on joints or spine. This set has been modernised to adapt to medical safety needs, so can be used in rehabilitation units and the likes.

The Author's Classes:
More information about the classes in Norfolk, England, run by the author of this book - Prof. Myke Symonds Shih-Jo - can be found at: www.TTTkungfu.com or on our Facebook pages: The Way of Heaven & earth School UK, Norwich T'ai Chi & Qigong for Health.

The author has also created other Facebook pages for the general public which have become very popular: Tao and Taoism in Britain Today. How to Get healthier & Loose Weight. Both free pages with lots of information and views on them.

CANCER
(Tumours)

Cancer is becoming more common and is increasingly associated with stress, pollutants (internal and external) and even drug side-effects. Tumours of other varieties may appear for different reasons, accidental damage to the brain area or suspect power source radiations, for example. However, the one thing that is emerging from scientific probing is that "negative thinking" is definitely not helping to cure tumours of any form. Is it possible that the dull, uninspiring atmosphere within many hospitals is not always encouraging either, overworked and tired looking staff, bless them, who may be stressed or unfit themselves? How can they hope to encourage patients to gird their loins and fight it when they are giving out negative signs? I try to be fair, and in some cases there are some excellent staff or helpers... but the system is overloaded. It is tied down with drugs and surgery being the *only* options and is considerably restricted by orthodox practices which, in my opinion, should be scrapped. All right, scanning and testing is of importance, I am not denying that. It is the treatment end that needs a radical shake up and inclusion of the better established, tried and tested Chinese techniques:

Facts.
In Chinese Hospitals they have adopted some Western practices and equipment. Generally though they have evaluated the use of drugs and found them to be of lesser value than Traditional Chinese Medicine (TCM) practises. Research using the latest methods has been finding some startling facts about TCM. For example, in many parts of the world deep breathing techniques have been associated with amazing healing, including the riddance of tumours. In China this exercise is called Ch'i Kung (Qigong) and has been formalised over the centuries into different exercises for different illnesses. There are also exercises for general health and well being. The most important aspect of Ch'i, often pronounced as "Qi", is that of energy; Qi-gong means "Energy training". Qi is the body's natural bio-energy, we all have it from conception and birth. Without it our body would die on us; like a car with a flat battery.

Wei Qi is the name used to describe part of the bio-energy that cannot only be built up in strength but "transmitted" out of the body and to someone else. In ignorance of the scientific facts, those who practice some form of "laying on of hands", like Spiritualists or Reiki

Practitioners, are actually transmitting their Wei Qi. Qi is formed as three major energy types, two of which are bio-magnetic and infra-red microwaves. Of the two, the latter is the most powerful healer, though in certain cases the bio-magnetism can be better. The hands, specifically the centre of the palms, are the best transmitters; though Qi can be sent out from any part of the body just about. An experienced Qigong Master can direct his Qi to the necessary area/s within a patient and effect healing processes that are safe, natural and far beyond any surgery or drugs. In my case I have "sensed" imbalances whilst sitting near people, standing at the front of a Taiji or Qigong class and even via greater distances. Some students and friends have been more than amazed by this; like Mary whom I telephoned one day and suggested that she checked her husband's Meridians (energy channels) on his chest for a point of imbalance. It was there.

Anyhow, back to the plot. The modern Chinese health authorities have commissioned many tests linked with Qi and Qigong. In 1980, for example, the Eighth People's Hospital in Shanghai Mr. Lin Housheng successfully applied Waiqi as an anaesthetic in surgery; nothing else was used, no acupuncture or drugs, just Qi directed by a well known Master.

FURTHER PROOF
Research institutes have discovered many amazing facts about Qigong and its effects on the human physiology and psychology; all of which have proven right the claims of the ancient Masters, incidentally. One such discovery is that the human immune system, with defensive and regenerative systems, is greatly enhanced by the practice of Qigong or Taijiquan, (this, as past Masters stated, is due to the effect which takes place within the blood and bone marrow). Waiqi has been found by medical scientists to be a low frequency modulated infra-red radiation. Mr. Lin, like some other Qigong and Internal Martial Arts practitioners can direct this energy from the palms of the hands or fingertips. In his series of experiments using Ch'i as anaesthetic in thyroidectomies, nine out of ten used only the permitted dose of 10 ml of externally applied local anaesthetic to the skin that was cut in the operations. One was carried out successfully even without this. Mr. Lin (of the Shanghai Traditional Chinese Medicine Research Institute) has had a great deal of success with cancer. The Waiqi has been shown through clinical experiments to kill cancer cells that are later discharged from the body and raises the degree of cancer immunity.

In 1986 under scientific conditions (December 19), Master Yen Xin demonstrated his ability to transmit his Ch'i over 2,000 Kilometres and change the molecular structure of different liquids. The experiment was conducted at the famous and highly respected Qing Hua University of Peking.

The problems that can arise from this kind of ability should not be overlooked, for people might say, "Why can't you heal everybody all over the world?" This is impossible, even for a huge army of healers. The people who utter these kind of rash questions should bear in mind that it is every individual's responsibility to look after themselves. A teacher is a teacher first and healer second. Those with whom personal contact is made can be helped and more importantly, shown how to help themselves through the Taoist Arts. The main principle of this book is to look at dietary functions, but as this topic of Qigong and cancer suggests, by taking up proper guided qi-gong exercises you can help yourself even further.

IMPORTANT NOTE

It is all right to recall such events, but what we must focus on is not the Art, skill, type of therapy or the person who administers it. The focus is on you, or other people who need help and advice. In the Chinese Arts we have many young students join us who may be looking for "secrets", short cuts and the "easy way" of training without all that long, hard work. There are no short cuts, no easy way. As we Shih-fu (teachers) say, "I cannot walk the Way for you. I am merely a signpost; I can point you in the right direction and say, 'there's the path'. You must make the efforts and walk that path yourself". It is the individuals who must help themselves. Every teacher, every healer, every person with skills has those skills because they made the efforts to learn and sustained those efforts over the years. In the affluent West, such as UK and USA, we are brought up to rely upon the orthodox medical system and go to them when we are ill. We are not taught how we can *prevent* illness by looking after ourselves, just how to crawl to the GP when we are already ill. The system undermines our need to look after ourselves properly.

Cancer, like many other illnesses, is telling us that we have neglected our well-being; we have not eaten correctly, reduced stress or thought wisely for some time, enough for the illness to develop. However, never say never, never say it is too late to change. Without hope we cannot build an image of how we would like to be, without a positive image we have no pattern to follow, no path to walk. Make your self a destiny and the path will be there.

CUT or CURE?

Orthodox Medicine has not made any real progress in the treatments of cancer for over thirty years, surgery remains virtually the same and chemotherapy or radiation is still used ad hoc. Many thousands of cancer sufferers are turning to other forms of treatment. Why? For a start there is an increase in the number of people who develop cancer every year. It is estimated that by the year 2000+ that 1-in-2 people will have some form of cancer at some time in their life, if nothing is done to prevent it; changes in food production, drink, environmental pollution, lifestyle, etcetera. It is a sad fact that for all the millions of pounds/dollars spent on cancer research that they have achieved very little. Some may say nothing valuable at all. At the same time thousands more people every year are turning to Traditional Medicine. Longer established techniques that are not "experimental", like common orthodox practises. Based on whatever principle, the tried and trusted treatments are established and do have a credible record. Of course, the thing that annoys Western Medical practitioners is that in many cases they cannot dissect it and put a name to the specific element that effects a cure or positive change. If they could, then some bright entrepreneur would try to sell it via a drug company in pill form, or pass themselves off as another "genius doctor invents new miracle cure and gets a Nobel prize"; all that happened was they gave it a name that nobody could understand or even associate with the original method or herb, etcetera.

If this all sounds a little bitter, then "yes", I own up, I am. Why should I not dislike such practises when they experiment with drugs and surgical techniques and try to justify their own presence; and super high salary or claims to fame. Every week on the news we hear of surgeons who kill "by error", drugs which have horrific and often deadly side-effects. A medical fact is that prescribed painkillers kill over 2,000 people a year. Heaven knows how many more die from over the counter bought painkillers! If I go to my family practitioner I want proper examination and proper enquiry with proper treatments, not a shrug and "Go home, take two aspirins and lay down. It might go away".

In his book, 'Fighting Cancer; a survival guide plus an a-z of cancer treatment options.', author Jonathan Chamberlain asks, "What is cancer? How we define the disease affects how we treat it. So we must ask ourselves: is the tumour the disease or is it a symptom of the disease? Do we concentrate on attacking the tumour or do we try to heal the body?" He adds, "Orthodox modern Western medicine considers the cancerous tumour to be the disease itself. How or why it arose they have no idea. But having arisen, it must be attacked... surgically removed. Or irradiated. Or killed with highly toxic chemicals... " etcetera. Having stated the orthodox view he states the traditional view, "Alternative medicine, on the other hand, posits that the tumour symptom will disappear once the root cause disappears." This "cause" is most often seen as the lack of care, improper diet or abuse of the body by drugs, chemicals and/or poisons.

His book quotes medical facts and facts of success and failures in attempts to heal or cure cancer. The book covers just about every aspect, types of treatments, cure rates and any doubtable methods backed up by facts. One thing that he stresses though is that whatever you choose it must be your choice (not a doctor's, surgeon's or therapist's or even a friend's), your choice with which you feel comfortable and happy. You need to have complete faith in what you are doing.

COMMON SYMPTOMS

- **Green undertone on one or both sides of the face • A solid lump (growing or static) • Unusual bleeding or discharge from any orifice • Sores which do not heal • Difficulty in swallowing (lump in throat) • Changes in warts or moles • Persistent coughing or hoarseness of throat • Persistent ache or nagging pain in a certain area •**
Persistent headaches or blinding pains • Unexplained changes in bowel or bladder movements •

Generally speaking it is hard to diagnose cancer *before* it becomes physically obvious. The Traditional Chinese Medicine approach is *avoid*. To do this we must look at those things that are commonly associated with cancer; smoking, diet - meat - carcinogens - drinks, pollution and negative attitude.

FIVE ELEMENT THEORY
This depends on the starting point. For example, it could be the lungs through smoking, or the gut through dietary abuse, the liver through

smoking and drinking alcohol, and so on. There are or may be many factors involved. The TCM theory remains one whereby the cancer is a symptom of impurity, of clogged and poisoned internal works. Therefore to treat the symptoms one must cleanse the system, replace the damaging factors (poisoning) of your lifestyle with those that are strengthening and building (healing) and develop a resolute will to change and be healthy again.

SMOKING

One out of two smokers will develop related diseases. Only fifteen percent of a cigarette is inhaled directly, out of the smoke that comes off there are over 4000 chemicals, at least 60 of these are known to cause cancer; smokers cause non-smokers to inhale these chemicals; murder by any other name. Smokers also inhale these chemicals as they hold their cigarettes. According to recent research, mothers who smoke can transfer many of the deadly toxic chemicals to their babies or children within two hours of smoking, just by being close to them or breathing near them. Carbon dioxide is another of the gasses that comes off a burning cigarette, it kills (the same gas which comes from vehicle exhausts). Others include, cadmium, arsenic, nicotine, hydrogen cyanide and ammonia. Manufacturers of cigarettes are killing people by the millions, a painful, slow and agonising death from an addictive drug.

According to a 1998 survey, only one in six women who smoke give up during pregnancy. The unborn baby is affected through the blood stream. To smoke, or intake anything else harmful whilst pregnant, will affect the unborn child's future health; this could include a premature and painful death. Even smoking and then quitting before pregnancy can have detrimental effects.

As this book goes to press there is a smoking ban imminent in public places in the England, this includes bars, Guest Houses, Shops and Factories. There are a few smokers still who adamantly refuse to give up and foolishly refute claims made concerning 'passive smoking'. All I can say about that is, if you are fool enough to suck smoke into your lungs – completely unnatural – then go somewhere deserted to inflict self-damage, like a desert island, but do not smoke near me!

FOOD FACTORS

Red meat has long been associated with such diseases. The common skin spots called 'moles' (brown spots) are said to be the effects of toxins from meat coming to the surface. Nowadays there are newer threats as food manufacturers turn to unproven methods of growing foods or adding ingredients, like aspartame or spraying vegetables with chemicals to kill common insects. There are so many foods involved here that it would be easier to just list the main items of doubt in the 'Foods To Avoid' section below. In this section I shall also include those items, such as aspartame, which scientists have expressed considerable doubt over. Also included will be other toxic substances that are inhaled or digested and are considered dangerous and/or possible causes of cancerous tumours.

All that I can add to this is to say that armed with the facts it is then your decision, your choice as to what to do about it. If you find yourself in a position, work environs for example, where you know or suspect that the atmosphere or food is suspect, then it is up you to do something about it. Never suffer in silence. Never accept anything which will damage your or other's health. Fight it and win. Remember what strength there is in numbers. If you find something on your local supermarket shelves which has a "dodgy" ingredient, leave it but turn the 'Ingredients:" list to face outwards, so that prospective buyers will at least be aware of the list and may look at it themselves. Too often manufacturers make the list so small, or hidden in a fold on a packet, that it cannot be easily seen. There again some manufacturers use loopholes in the laws to "group" certain questionable ingredients under another name or phrase. Write to supermarkets and complain about such products or practises, or anything that may contain unhealthy items. Fight it. Make it change. You are the consumer, without your support, your purchase, your approval (silent or otherwise) they have no power over you, they cannot do whatever it is that is offensive or dangerous in practice.

The law seemingly is designed to protect industrialists; who may often have board members involved in governmental affairs. If they produce foodstuffs which cause illness or death (just look at the CJD and "Mad Cow" disease debacle) they can get away Scott free. If you deliberately poisoned another person you would be prosecuted for murder or even manslaughter if you were proven to be "unaware" of the outcome! Change it. It is your choice, you either allow it to happen or fight for fair changes.

FOODS TO BE AVOIDED.

MEAT: Blue (shark, mackerel, etcetera), red (beef, pork/ham/bacon, fowl), salmon and tuna, etcetera. Also, chicken/turkey may carry up to twice the levels of bacteria than animal meats.

ANIMAL PRODUCE: especially those high in cholesterol and fats (eggs, dairy cream, chocolates, full fat cheese, butter, yoghurt, bacon fat).

FATS: Whilst Soya (beans/milk/oil, etcetera) produce has been recommended for those suffering from cancer, ask for "de-fatted soya" products. Soya fat is high and high fat induces heart disease as well.

SUGAR: White "refined" sugar or anything it is added to. Artificial sweeteners. Cut back on all sweeteners including honey or raw cane sugars.

ALCOHOL: No spirits. Little wine. Moderate beers; especially women.

These are the main foods associated with cancer so far. Modern research has implicated all of the above with tumours and most with heart disease. There are many reports and surveys that implicate fatty foods, especially meat and animal produce. Further research will no doubt prove more specific.

OTHER THINGS TO AVOID:

PILLS: The birth control pill. Strong drugs.
SMOKING: All smoking is harmful and kills.
CHEMICALS: Workplace, household sprays, garden sprays, dips or fumes; especially exhaust fumes, petrol or diesel.
ELECTRICAL FIELDS: There is growing concern about electromagnetic fields (EMF's) in many areas; radio, mobile phones, electric blankets, coils in heaters, toasters, kettles, etcetera. There is great concern for those who live under or very near power lines or buried cables.
EXCESS DIETARY FIBRE: We need regular amounts of natural dietary fibre, but some people go too far and consume extra roughage (perhaps cereal based), which has been related to colonic cancer cases. Moderation in all things.

NITRATES: Pickled and "smoked" foods. They contain large amounts of nitrates that are easily converted to a highly potent class of carcinogenic chemicals called Nitrosamines.

TRAUMA: Many cancer patients have undergone physical trauma (post accidental damage) or severe mental stresses. Whilst accidents cannot always be avoided (more care can be taken!), stress can nearly always be avoided or reduced.

VIRUSES: One third of cancer cases are thought to be caused by viruses. It is believed that these unknown viruses may change appearance between virus and bacteria, so remaining "hidden" better. However, keeping the immune system well by looking after yourself will eliminate many viruses.

SUPPORTIVE FOODS.

Pulses: Beans, lentils and peas (Legumes).
Dairy: Soya milk or cheese (low fat vegetable or de-fatted), goat's milk cheese.
Meat: not advised generally but cod or haddock (white fish from deep sea).
Nuts: Roasted peanuts in shells, Brazil nuts, walnuts.
Vegetables: Broccoli, cauliflower, cabbage, Brussels sprouts; these have been shown to have anti-mutagenic properties.
Grains: Buckwheat, barley, millet, rice (brown, short grain).
Fruits: Fresh fruits that are local and in season, natural dried fruits.
Oils: *Sunflower oil, "Pure" and margarine (avoid impure brands).
Drinks: Ban Cha (green tea), herbal teas, mountain spring water, dandelion coffee, unsweetened fruit juices (but *not* acidic "citrus" fruits, including orange), vegetable juices and or vegetable stocks.
Flour: Corn cakes/flour, oats/oat cakes, millet, rice flour, rye and rye crisp breads, tofu.

*Detail: Researchers across the world have found that decreasing red meats and fatty foods will help reduce risk of cancer. At the same time, an increase or change to more fresh vegetables, fresh fruit and (de-fatted) soya products will help protect against cancer; except those cancers caused by smoking or other chemical influence.

Colonic cancer risk in particular is lessened by the intake of high fibre, especially fibre that comes from vegetables, specialists say. As we have already seen in other illnesses caused by a bad diet, leafy green vegetables come to the rescue, so to speak.

High calorific content and fatty diets, red meats (beef, pork, lamb, etc), all appear to increase the risk of colonic cancer and possibly other "gut" cancers. There have been conflicting reports on the effect of saturated fat. Some studies have suggested that it is "an important risk factor", not to be overlooked, while others have shown no effect or even a protective effect. This variance must surely be caused by the individual's genes. Some cancer research specialists have said that they have found some generic links to cancer, these being triggered by food, pollution or other environmental factors.

HYPOGLYCAEMIA
Low or plummeting Blood Sugar

Hypoglycaemia is more common than you might at first think. Many who suffer from the illness are never diagnosed; others may be incorrectly diagnosed as 'neurotic' or suffering from mental stress. There are three types of hypoglycaemic symptoms:

(1) Severe hypoglycaemia: This may result from organic disease, such as insulin producing tumours of the pancreas. The condition is dangerous and coma could result from sugar loss. Fatal unless cleared.

(2) Diabetic hypoglycaemia: May occur when someone is already diabetic and has to administer their own doses of insulin. If the insulin is overdosed their blood sugar levels may drop dramatically causing blackouts or other problems.

(3) Reactive hypoglycaemia: Sometimes called 'rebound hypoglycaemia" is less dangerous than the other two and is caused by metabolic dysfunctions. It is most common among women and can have very destructive effects on the lives of the sufferers and their friends, families or work associates, especially under stressful conditions.

COMMON SYMPTOMS
- **Allergic reactions** • **Anxiety** • **Behavioural problems and mood swings** • **Cold sweats** • **Epilepsy (but only in those who are susceptible)** • **Fainting or feeling faint** • **Fast Heart beat (tachocardia)**
- **Headaches** • **Hunger or nausea** • **Insomnia (possible 'sleep walking' or 'midnight snacking'** • **Irritability** • **Memory problems** • **Migraines**
- **Palpitations** • **Period problems** • **Personality disorders (including hysteria and/or hypochondriasis)** • **Selfishness ("I need ..." behaviour, inconsideration of partner/friends)** • **Stress intolerance** • **Vertigo** • **Water reactions (mucus)** • **Weakness (trembling limbs or feeling weak).**

FIVE ELEMENT THEORY
The pancreas normally controls the blood sugar within very fine limits. If the blood sugar is consistently too high the person may become

diabetic, too low and they become hypoglycaemic. The pancreas produces the hormone 'insulin' which drives the glucogen into the cells resulting in the fall of blood sugar and the symptoms. The effect is worsened if the sufferer eats sugary snacks (cakes, biscuits, sweets, chocolate, etcetera.), especially on an empty stomach. The sugar enters the blood stream really quickly, just as quickly the pancreas is stimulated into releasing insulin. As the insulin drives the blood sugar into the cells it leaves the blood depleted. One of the most common symptoms occurs as the blood sugar levels drop for there is not enough glucose to feed the brain; the first organ to be affected. This leads to confused or muddled thinking (blaming others for one's own decisions/thinking that people are conspiring against them, etcetera), aggressive outbursts (blaming others/'having a go' at others for no apparent reason to those concerned), feelings of uncertainty, memory retention problems, sudden mood swings and depressions. Obviously these symptoms may not be 'felt' or recognised by the sufferer but may be living hell for those who are involved with them. Friends or colleagues may 'stand accused' for no reason, or shouted at for no apparent reason, blamed for things that they have not done or pushed away because of unfounded fears of the sufferer. For the sufferers this poses a problem as they may not recognise these symptoms, as may be the case with friends, colleagues and families of course. Help should be sought.

Other symptoms such as fainting, trembling or shaking, weakness of the limbs, dizziness, strange behaviour, selfish behaviour, frequent headaches, fatigue and various skin disorders, rashes or allergies are all very common. Combinations of these would warrant a trip to a GP to get the blood sugar levels checked.

In dietary terms the condition may be caused by a lacking of certain vitamins or minerals whilst eating too many sugary foods. On a broader scale it may also be viewed by TCM (Traditional Chinese Medicine) as an emotionally based problem with physical repercussions, The Spleen/Pancreas Meridian (energy channel) is the most obviously affected with probable symptoms being detected with the Heart, Lung and Liver Meridians. At certain times or under certain conditions there may be detectable imbalances of the Stomach, Small and Large Intestines and the Kidney Meridians. The spleen is responsible for storing blood for emergencies as well as 'recycling' the blood. The liver (which has over 500 functions) also acts as a (delete 'an emergency') reservoir of blood for emergencies and filters the blood ridding it of unwanted toxins, etcetera. If the liver is damaged by either excess or deficiencies then various reactions including allergies may be seen. Symptoms occur frequently and may follow vigorous exercise, eating sweet foods or condensed fruit drinks, etcetera. Being a condition linked to the Spleen/Pancreas Meridian 'dampness' will effect the problems. Work or sports associated with water (surfing, windsurfing, water skiing, rafting, sailing, swimming, car wash spray or similar, foggy weather or damp conditions) can all aggravate symptoms. Vigorous exercise will burn off blood sugar too quickly and often the sufferer will feel the desire to eat 'quick energy' foods, such as sugary biscuits, to get a burst of energy. This must be avoided as it will give a burst of energy for ten or so minutes but will stimulate the pancreas to produce insulin which will then drive the glucogen into the cells and cause a longer lasting 'down' effect. Because of these sudden swings the sufferers can appear to be neurotic, temperamental and unpredictable. Stressful work or stressful relationships will all contribute to bringing on the symptomatic swings. Chinese Arts such as T'ai Chi Ch'uan (Taiji Quan) and Ch'i Kung (Qigong) can help reduce symptoms by lowering the metabolic rate; only if practised over a long period of time and daily. These are not 'stand alone' and should be done in conjunction with a vitamin and mineral supplement as well as support from a partner (if possible) who can help 'monitor' daily effects; Hypoglycaemia sufferers by nature of the illness may not recognise the symptoms due to the effects on the brain activity. Coming full circle again, food is a major key and a strict dietary regime should be adhered to. The proper diet is not difficult to follow at home but problems are likely to occur when eating out. Food should be chosen very carefully.

FOOD FACTORS
Western orthodox nutritional medicine recognises *some* of the most common causal foods: e.g. dairy produce and refined carbohydrates.

These are responsible for more than just hypoglycaemia and can be partially responsible for other common diseases such as asthma and sinusitis. It is also thought that under activity of the thyroid gland may be partially responsible as it contributes to blood sugar and hence energy levels. The thyroid gland is the only part of the human body that uses iodine in regular daily doses in its function. Iodine may be found in salt, but salt must not be over used. If in any doubt then a regular daily supplement can be taken and is much safer than taking extra salt. Excess iodine will be flushed out of the system.

FOODS TO BE AVOIDED
Avoid all refined carbohydrates (white flour, white sugar, icing sugar, white rice, in cakes, tea, sweets, biscuits, et cetera.),
Alcohol, coffee and tea.
Raw foods and juices (especially during autumn and winter months).
Tropical or citrus fruits and drinks (unless you are living in the tropics or countries where they are local).
Concentrated fruit drinks.
Any food or drink with added glucose, fructose or sugars. Fatty foods.
Meats.
Dairy produce (unless low fat and in moderation).
Roasted nuts.
Yeast or yeast extracts.

SUPPORTIVE FOODS
Warm foods and those foods with added cinnamon, cardamom, ginger, ginseng and nutmeg, lemon and fennel.
Aduki and kidney beans (WARNING: Kidney beans should be soaked overnight and well cooked before eating!).
Millet; gluten free so it does not create mucus (soak overnight then rinse well several times, cook for exactly ten minutes).
Late summer root vegetables: Sweet potatoes, squashes (zucchini), parsnips, carrots and turnips, corn (maize) alfalfa, barley, celery, mustard, garlic and onions, horseradish.
All leafy green vegetables (in season preferably) and broccoli. Fresh parsley.
Black pepper and cayenne pepper in moderation.
Walnuts, pistachio nuts.
Black dates (help replenish Spleen Ch'i).
Chicken (organic only).

Foods that lower blood sugar and give support to the spleen/pancreas: Artichokes, Brussels sprouts, buckwheat, cucumber (stir fried), garlic, green beans, oats, onions, soya beans or soya products (de-fatted), legumes and pulses. Do not eat too many of these in one meal, try to balance the foods out. If you eat locally grown, seasonal fruit then lightly stewed is best as this warms the food.

COMPLEX CARBOHYDRATES (Can be good for you!)
- Barley • Buckwheat • Millet • Potatoes (baked, boiled or low fat

sunflower oil, oven chips • **Oats** • Short grain brown rice • Whole wheat • Yams.

GINGER
The great healer: although some people in Orthodox Medicine deny this nowadays. In China if anyone is suffering from injury, illness or cold symptoms (other than 'fever') ginger is added to teas and soups. It has a warming effect and therefore wards off cold and dampness. If having a salad, which has 'cold' leafy green vegetables and other salad foods, then it is advisable to add a pinch of ginger to the salad dressing. Another tip is to have a baked potato with the salad, the hot and dry (Yang) counter-balancing the cold/damp (Yin) foods.

ALCOHOL
It may produce temporary relief from symptoms but could become habitual and therefore damage the liver. Those who are recovering from alcoholism should also take the vitamin and mineral supplements of the hypoglycaemic recovery regime.

FOOD SUPPLEMENTS
• Apricots • Blue-green algae • Spirulina • Eggs or egg yolk • Figs • Nettles or nettle tea • Lycii ("Lychee") berries • Sardines or other 'oily fish'.

GLYCERINE
A vegetable extract often used in food production or cooking. It may be obtained from a chemist and in small doses at very rare intervals may help those who suffer from hypoglycaemia symptoms such as waking during the early hours of the morning. Some sufferers have found that one teaspoonful of glycerine will help them get off to sleep. It does this by gently boosting the blood sugar levels. However, this is only a poor temporary measure and should not be relied upon. Personally I would not recommend it. Deep breathing exercises will oxygenate the brain and induce better sleep. A corrective diet will also supply the right nutrients and the vitamin and mineral supplements help too.

SMOKING (Direct and 'passive' smoking)
Cigarette, pipe and cigar smoking will aggravate hypoglycaemia. Generally, smoking will contaminate the body with nicotine and tar, cause blood circulation problems and possible heart attacks or cancer. The effects are most noticeable on the lungs at first where the tar blocks

the delicate membranous fibres that the oxygen should pass through into the blood stream. Knock-on effects will cause problems with the pancreas, spleen and liver as well as general blood conditions.

EXERCISE

Regular exercise can improve blood sugar levels and regulate the metabolic system. Oxygen is essential for building and repairing every Cell in the body, as well as other more obvious functions. If new to exercise then it should be started slowly and gently, just one or two days per week. Gradually the exercises may be built up to three or four days per week and increased in terms of effort. As stated above, T'ai Chi Ch'uan (Taijiquan) and Ch'i Kung (Qigong) are very good forms of exercise for regulating and lowering the metabolic rate, but they are not 'stamina' exercises. Any exercise which is fast or vigorous will require large amounts of energy, so the diet must be tailored accordingly and extra 'energy foods' (complex carbohydrates, starches, food sugars, proteins, amino acids, Vitamin B_3 and oxygen are the essential components).

REST

Those who are hypoglycaemic may be physically exhausted. Try to eat properly and sleep only at the proper times. Waking at night time can mean that sufferers become exhausted during the day and disruptive patterns are set up (see glycerine below).

STRESS

A stressful job or family situation can be a triggering factor or the stress could also be a result of hypoglycaemia. If in a stressful job then try to change it for one in which stress levels are far less. Squabbling families or rowing partners, coping by ones self and 'dashing around' between work and play whilst missing meals is all very stressful, as is travelling and all that goes with it. Coming home to a calming environment is also very beneficial, as is having a helpful partner/family and friends who not only understand but can help by their 'recognition' of symptoms and times of need as well as encouragement or support where proper eating is concerned.

HYPERVENTILATION

Uncontrollable over-breathing can make the management of hypoglycaemia very difficult. It will make worse current symptoms. Again Qi Gong and Taiji can help here by regulating the breath as well as lowering the metabolic rate so that the body's management system works at a more even pace.

DRUGS

Metronidazole, prescribed for the treatment of vaginal trichmoniasis, has been found to cause hypoglycaemic symptoms. Anyone who experiences any hypoglycaemic symptoms whilst on drug treatments should bear in mind that the drug is creating the symptoms by means of the side-effects, or less directly by lowering blood sugar levels. If in doubt consult your GP, a specialist or appropriate health therapist.

GENERAL ADVICE

- Do not miss or skip meals • Breakfast is the most important meal of the day. Organic oats (for porridge) may be soaked overnight to facilitate easier cooking in the morning (five minutes in a microwave oven!). Muesli is another beneficial as long as it is organic.
- Other meals should be of good protein value •
- Avoid all processed foods and refined carbohydrates •
- High complex carbohydrates are good for you`• (see above).
- If you are in a hurry it will only take approximately ten minutes to microwave cook a 'baking' potato (five minutes each side). It can be cooked while you are getting other things ready and can be accompanied by a wide range of healthy foods.
- Avoid all sweets, sticky buns, cakes and things containing white sugar (jams, cakes, chocolates, icing sugars and such like).

VITAMINS & MINERAL SUPPLEMENTS (Check with Specialist)

B - complex (B1, 2, 3, 6, 12); 20 -100 mg (milligram) per day.
Vitamin C; 2000 - 3000 mg per day minimum.
Chromium GTF; 200 mg per day (otherwise 200 mcg of Chromium Chloride in the formulae of 'CrCl3' which can be made up by your chemist.
Manganese; 5 - 10 mg per day.
Potassium; 500 - 1000 mg per day minimum.

Trytophan; 500 - 1500 mg per day (with a complex carbohydrate diet).[1]
Those who suffer from hypoglycaemia may be prone to the following:
• Adrenalin - high levels of, through sport and/or work which is stressful.

---

[1] Zen comes from the Chinese Ch'an, a mixture of Buddhist, Confucian and Taoist philosophies with no fixed form or preconceived plans; a kind of 'freestyle' enlightenment which often uses paradoxical statements to induce the thinking processes.

- Alcohol consumption over the recommended daily amount.
- Atopy (inherited tendency to allergies)
- Cholesterol; too high a blood count or intake.
- Diabetes or hypoglycaemia (blood sugar levels too high or low).
- Fats; too high an intake through meats, pastries, dairy foods, cakes, etc.

Other people that are not hypoglycaemic may suffer from such symptoms because of deficiencies in magnesium, zinc and B6. Deficiencies in essential fatty acids can cause problems in the metabolism of fatty acids into prostaglandin. Symptoms include;

- Blood clotting.
- Premenstrual Syndrome; especially where breast pain occurs.
- Dry eyes (most times but especially during sleep).
- Eczema, dry and itchy skin or psoriasis.
- Inflammation (All types, including arthritis).
- Migraines and headaches (on regular basis).

HYPERGLYCAEMIA.
Hyperglycaemia is a term used for High Blood Sugar Levels. This is often a problem associated with those who have Diabetes, Type 1 or 2, or pregnant women.

A person with Diabetes or Hyperglycaemia needs to keep their blood sugar levels at a constant and steady level, so avoid sugar binging, sweets or 'sins', as sweet treats are called these days.

Symptoms of Hyperglycaemia
Symptoms in people with diabetes tend to develop slowly over a few days or weeks. In some cases, there may be no symptoms until the blood sugar level is very high.

Symptoms of hyperglycaemia include:

- increased thirst and a dry mouth
- needing to pee frequently
- tiredness
- blurred vision
- unintentional weight loss

recurrent infections, such as thrush, bladder infections (cystitis) and skin infections: which could also be caused by other problems, so do get checked out.

Symptoms of hyperglycaemia can also be due to undiagnosed diabetes, so see your GP if this applies to you. You can have a simple test to check for the condition.

What causes high blood sugar?
A variety of things can trigger an increase in blood sugar level in people with diabetes, including:

- stress
- an illness, such as a cold
- eating too much, such as snacking between meals
- a lack of exercise
- dehydration
- missing a dose of your diabetes medication, or taking an incorrect dose over-treating an episode of hypoglycaemia (low blood sugar)
- Certain medicines, such as steroid medication.

Occasional episodes of hyperglycaemia can also occur in children and young adults during growth spurts.

Foods to Avoid:
You may be advised to:

- change your diet – for example, you may be advised to avoid foods that cause your blood sugar levels to rise, such as cakes or sugary drinks
- drink plenty of sugar-free fluids – this can help if you're dehydrated
- exercise more often – gentle, regular exercise such as walking can often lower your blood sugar level, particularly if it helps you lose weight
- if you use insulin, adjust your dose – your care team can give you specific advice about how to do this

You may also be advised by a GP to monitor your blood sugar level more closely, or test your blood or urine for substances called ketones (associated with diabetic ketoacidosis).

Until your blood sugar level is back under control, watch out for additional symptoms that could be a sign of a more serious condition, such as noted here.

Contact your diabetes care team immediately if you have a high blood sugar level and experience the following symptoms:

- feeling sick or being sick
- abdominal pains - it is not 'normal' to have pains
- rapid, deep breathing but not from exercise
- signs of dehydration, such as a headache, dry skin and a weak, rapid heartbeat
- difficulty staying awake

These symptoms could be a sign of diabetic ketoacidosis or a hyperosmolar hyperglycaemic state (see above) and you may need to be looked after in hospital.

Hyperglycaemia sounds similar to Hypoglycaemia but can be more life or health damaging and needs to be treated with care.

Irritable Bowel Syndrome (IBS)

Irritable Bowel Syndrome is very common in the west. Doctors of orthodox medicine tend to view it as a mixture of symptoms that they believe to be caused by a disorder of the intestinal motor function (food processing and transportation: food is moved along the gut by a series of muscular contractions, thus causing the intestines to be systematically "squeezed" and thus propelling the ingested food along the channel). There are also areas within the intestines where the process slows down and the food is held whilst processing takes place, this is called segmentation. This combination of propulsion and segmentation is called peristalsis. When the system is working normally, one is completely unaware of it.

EAST
The China Health Project
The China Project on Nutrition, Health & Environment is a massive study involving researchers from China, Cornell University in Ithaca, New York, and the University of Oxford, into the relationships between diet, lifestyles and disease-related mortality in 6500 Chinese subjects from 65 mostly rural or semi-rural counties.

The rural Chinese diet is largely vegetarian or vegan, and involves less total protein, less animal protein, less total fat and animal fat, and more carbohydrate and fibre than the average Western diet. Blood cholesterol levels are significantly lower. Heart disease, cancer, obesity, diabetes, and osteoporosis are all uncommon. Areas in which they are becoming more frequent are areas where the population has moved towards a more Western diet with increasing consumption of animal products.

The China Health Project has clearly demonstrated the health benefits of a diet based on plant foods. One of the Project's co-ordinators, Dr Colin Campbell of Cornell University, has stated that, "We're basically a vegetarian species and should be eating a wide variety of plant foods and minimising our intake of animal foods." (Source: The China Health Project website)

WEST

Western doctors believe that, "In addition to the intestinal symptoms, psychological factors are commonly involved", which is completely unfounded. It is however more likely that stress (a mental health symptom) can be part cause of IBS. In the UK about 14 per cent of women and 6 per cent of men suffer from Irritable Bowel Syndrome. According to data published on the Internet, "Although the cause is unknown, about half of all patients will date the onset of their symptoms to a major life event such as change of house or job, or bereavement. This suggests that there may be a psychological (possibly stress) trigger in susceptible patients. Approximately 10 to 20 per cent of patients will date the onset of their symptoms to an acute gastroenteritis. In the remainder, the trigger factor remains unidentified."

Common Symptoms
Symptoms may vary from person to person. Nerve-signalling chemicals, particularly serotonin, appear to have an important role, this may be caused by dietary intake as well as digestive malfunction.

Symptoms of the Oesophagus ('Adams Apple' - Upper throat)
• A sensation which feels "like a golf ball in the throat" but not interfering with swallowing (globus). • Heartburn - burning pain often felt behind the breastbone.
• Painful swallowing (odynophagia), but without hold-up of food. • Sticking of food (dysphagia) - this requires medical investigation.

Symptoms of the Stomach (below the heart)
• Non-ulcer dyspepsia (symptoms which may be suggestive of a stomach or duodenal ulcer, but which has not been confirmed on medical investigation). • Feeling full after small meals. This may also reach the stage of not being able to finish a meal. • Abdominal bloating after meals.

Symptoms of the Small Bowel (Stomach area)
• Increased gurgling noises which may be loud enough to cause social embarrassment (borborygmi). • Abdominal bloating; can be so severe that women describe themselves as looking pregnant. • Generalised

abdominal tenderness associated with bloating. • Abdominal bloating of both types usually subsides overnight and returns the following day.

Symptoms of the Large Bowel (Abdominal)

• Abdominal bloating of both types usually subsides overnight and returns the following day. • Right-sided abdominal pain, either low, or tucked up under the right ribs. Does not always get better on opening the bowels. • Pain tucked up under the left ribs (splenic flexure syndrome). • When the pain is bad, it may enter the left armpit. • Variable and erratic bowel habits alternating from constipation to diarrhoea. • Increased gastro-colic reflex. This is an awakening of the childhood reflex where food in the stomach stimulates colonic activity, resulting in the need to open the bowels. • Severe, short stabbing pains in the rectum, called proctalgia fugax.

Symptoms of Other functions or organs

• Headaches are common. • In women, left-sided abdominal pain on sexual intercourse is not uncommon. • Increased frequency of passing urine is common. • Fatigue and tiredness are very common.
• Sleep disturbance is also frequent.
• Loss of appetite is common, as is nausea. • Features of depression occur in about one third of patients. • Anxiety and stress-related symptoms are common and may interact with the gut symptoms.

Orthodox medicine does not offer at this time any insight into clarification of symptoms that should *not* be accredited to irritable bowel syndrome.

The NHS say:
"It's usually a lifelong problem. It can be very frustrating to live with and can have a big impact on your everyday life.

> **•There's no cure, but diet changes and medicines can often help control the symptoms.**
>
> **•The exact cause is unknown** – it's been linked to things like food passing through your gut too quickly or too slowly, oversensitive nerves in your gut, stress and a family history of IBS."

The symptoms are:
• Difficulty in swallowing when food gets stuck. • Indigestion-type pain that wakes the patient at night. • Abdominal bloating which does not get better overnight. • Significant and unexplained weight loss. • The presence of bleeding from the back passage. • Chronic, painless diarrhoea.

Generally one should get medical consultation and (if necessary, such as in the case of rectal bleeding or blood in the stools) thorough examination and tests. Do not procrastinate, as internal disorders can be serious. At the same time, do not be alarmed to the extent of seeking surgery if other cures have not been tried, like dietary correction and prescribed exercises, et cetera.

Foods to be Avoided
As stated above, it is usually found that in places where the diet is predominantly non-meat and dairy foods that there is virtually a lack of IBS, as well as other common diseases found in the west or places with "westernised" diets.

My suggestions based on the research that has gone into this book from various specialist sources are:

• **Meats** • **Alcohol** • **Coffee** • **Dairy Foods (milk, cream, butter, etc.)** • **Fatty Foods (includes full fat Soya!)** • **High Protein Diets** • **Spicy Foods** •

Other factors to be avoided:
• **Large Meals** • **Meals after 7 pm** • **Lack of Exercise** • **Slumped Posture at Work or Home** • **Stressful Situations** • **Hurrying Food (Chew thoroughly).**

Foods which Help
• **Carbohydrates** • **Higher Fibre (increased gradually so that your stomach can get used to it!)** • **Balanced Intake (Carb's, vegetables, proteins and fruits)** • **Water (drink little and often)**

Other Helpful Factors
Food & Mood
Keep a daily 'food and mood diary' in which you make notes about which foods seem to upset your stomach, how long after a meal, the

state of your mind or feelings (e.g. mood swings, elation, depression, bowel movements, et cetera.

Exercise

Obviously exercise will help. We are creatures with bones, muscles and internal organs which all rely on the flow of blood and oxygen. Lack of exercise will always lead to pathogens. Taking up some gentle exercises are very enjoyable; much more so than sitting around feeling uncomfortable! T'ai Chi Ch'uan is a really great way of bringing on better internal health without strain; although one should take it seriously and do the exercises regularly, like twice a day for at least one hour each time. The benefits are outstanding. Like meditation, T'ai Chi Ch'uan (Taijiquan) is very calming and can relieve the stress of every day life.

Going for long walks, preferably in the countryside where the greenery will help relax you. A stroll along a quiet beach, possibly with your dog, or a good friend. Generally avoid stressful situations, like shopping centres and places that are too busy. If you are reasonably fit and have no heart condition, back problems or other limiting debilities, why not consider badminton, Frisbee, swimming and even some gentle yoga as alternating exercises: if you have any doubts about your health consult a competent physician first!

You're Getting Warmer!
Heat treatment with hot gel packs, hot-water bottles or carefully used electric blankets may also help to relieve the symptoms. It will not cure them though, as drugs or painkillers may not either.

One thing you do not want to do is to worry about your health. Worry is negative and can in itself lead to pathogens. Just try to enjoy life as much as possible, generating better energy and a happier environment. If you find this difficult then perhaps you should seriously consider trying to change your lifestyle.

Is Medicine and Antibacterial Agents Killing You?

Quote:
"If you know me, then you've heard me preach a thousand times not to live in an antibacterial world. Your immune system works well and it needs a job. Humans are all too eager to pop antibiotics when ill."
by FBRadmin | Aug 19, 2014

Link:
https://fbresearch.org/antibiotics-overuse-and-damaging-your-immune-system/

VIRUS – Corona (Covid) or other Virus and Colds.

Eat To beat Covid!

What Is 'Coronavirus'?
Coronavirus first emerged in the mid-1960's and there are seven different main versions of the virus broken into four groups: alpha, beta, gamma, and delta: over 14,000 Strains.

Common human coronavirus.
229E, NL63, OC43 & HKU1.

Other human coronavirus.
MERS-CoV (the beta coronavirus that causes Middle East Respiratory Syndrome, or MERS)

SARS-CoV (the beta coronavirus that causes severe acute respiratory syndrome, or SARS)

SARS-CoV-2 (the novel coronavirus that causes coronavirus disease 2019, or COVID-19).

Many of these strands are present in upper and lower respiratory infections and therefore are common. SARS-CoV was first reported in the early 2000's. It has only recently been introduced to the human population. That is to say it is not *new*, just new to humans. Other strands such as HKU1 and NL63 are present in many upper and lower respiratory infections. The first cultured human coronavirus (B814) was obtained from a boy with a typical Common Cold in 1965 and research and studies from that point on continued to find the virus mutating and appearing in different forms with various, but often similar, symptoms such as nasal congestion, fever and coughing.

SARS-CoV is the most aggressive version of coronavirus and in 2003, it killed 800 people. That was just almost unseen a forerunner of what was to come regarding the potential of mutating coronavirus and the effect it could have on the world as we have been seeing during the so-called Pandemic. The term "so-called" has been used as there are many, many Doctors, PhD Scientists in Microbiology, Virology and other "ology's" who say that Covid-19 is/was not as harmful as the normal Flu Virus, which kill more people every year.

The November 2019 through winter 2020 outbreak was a newly recorded variant of Coronavirus, hence named 'Covid-19'. Where and how it started is in great contention but I was told by a GP that the first cases here (Norfolk, UK) were recorded November 19th 2019. It has very heavy effects on breathing and lungs: *especially* if your Immune System is not operating at peak health! (Note: The Author had it November 2019 and it affected over 3.5 million adults in the UK.)

Coronavirus are a group of viruses that are common to mankind, Humans. They cause illnesses such as the common cold, to far more severe conditions such as Pneumonia, Middle East Respiratory Syndrome (MERS) and Severe Acute Respiratory syndrome (SARS). According to experts, outbreaks are quite common and there have been seven major outbreaks world-wide of Coronavirus Diseases.

The Symptoms.
The main symptoms of the new strain include:
* respiratory symptoms (lungs & airways) like Common Cold.
* fever - high temperature of 38.7 C or above.
* continuous or persistent dry cough.
* shortness of breath & breathing difficulties.
* loss of taste or smell.

In severe cases it is thought by some that the Covid-19 variant can cause Pneumonia, SARS (a severe form of Pneumonia), kidney failure and even death. However, the more severe cases appear to be amongst the 25% minority who already have what they call "pre-existing health conditions", such as Heart problems, Lungs, Obesity or Diabetes.

The world-wide survival rate has been stated at around 98% to 98.5% approximately, some say 99.1%. There has been a very big "bone of contention" between the Scientists the UK Gov, and others have used, and the less 'gagged' experts world-wide who have shown sincere concern. The panic caused by the mainstream news and media has concentrated *only* on the deaths, *not* the 98+% survivors or even those who have avoided it, or only had mild symptoms.

Testing for Covid-19.
This has raised many concerns around the world. The original method of testing was existent, but quite slow. This was AH-PCR. PCR stands for Polymerase Chain Reaction.

According to Daniel D. Rhoads, MD, the section head of Microbiology at Cleveland Clinic, "there are a couple of ways to detect SARS-CoV-2, the virus that causes COVID-19. Some tests look for a piece of the coating of the virus, or 'spikes' - they're called antigen tests - and other tests detect nucleic acid (such as RNA) belonging to the coronavirus.

RNA tests are highly sensitive. "These tests can remain positive even after somebody is no longer sick and no longer shedding virus that can infect other people, Antigen tests, by contrast, are generally quick and cheap but often less accurate than RNA tests for detecting the Novel Coronavirus. The problem is that antigen testing is more prone to false negative results, meaning these tests are more likely to miss cases of active infection. And neither antigen nor RNA testing predicts when someone is no longer contagious", says Dr. Rhoads.

The "Swab test", introduced in Spring 2020, is generally the one which many Medical professionals are concerned about. To keep it in simple terms, we all carry Covid virus, or fragments of past Covid Virus. These reside in particular in the back of the throat or nose, where the Swab tests are taken from. The PCR Test can pick up these "spikes" and even if "dead or non-active" virus, can label it as a "Positive Test", or "infectious". This is what they call a "False Positive". The concerns of the many experts are that these False Positives are being treated as Infectious, causing medical staff to hospitalise the patient, and therefore overloading the medical system, causing fear and panic and, worst of all, allowing the Government to implement unnecessary 'Lock-downs' on an unprecedented scale which are causing mass unemployment, mass mental and physical health problems and shutting down businesses, so ruining the economy too. The UK Government has been advised by these 'free' professionals but has chosen to ignore the advice in favour of their own select group of individuals: who do not appear to be anywhere near as "expert" as the others, world-wide.

Dr. Mike Yeadon, a former Vice President and Chief Science Officer for Pfizer for 16 years, says that half or even "almost all" of tests for COVID are false positives. Dr. Yeadon also argues that the threshold for herd immunity may be much lower than previously thought, and may have been reached in many countries already.

An article published by The Lancet (medical journal, England), September 29th 2020, states:

"RT-PCR tests to detect severe acute respiratory syndrome coronavirus 2 (SARS-CoV-2) RNA are the operational gold standard for detecting COVID-19 disease in clinical practice. RT-PCR assays in the UK have analytical sensitivity and specificity of greater than 95%, but no single gold standard assay exists. New assays are verified across panels of material, confirmed as COVID-19 by multiple testing with other assays, together with a consistent clinical and radiological picture. These new assays are often tested under idealised conditions with *hospital samples containing higher viral loads than those from asymptomatic individuals living in the community*. As such, diagnostic or operational performance of swab tests in the real world might differ substantially from the analytical sensitivity and specificity."

It continues on to say, "The current rate of operational false-positive swab tests in the UK is unknown; preliminary estimates show it could be somewhere between 0·8% and 4·0%. This rate could translate into a significant proportion of false-positive results daily due to the current low prevalence of the virus in the UK population, adversely affecting the positive predictive value of the test.
2 Considering that the UK National Health Service employs 1.1 million health-care workers, many of whom have been exposed to COVID-19 at the peak of the first wave, the potential disruption to health and social services due to false positives could be considerable."

(Download the PDF for yourself, if still available: https://www.thelancet.com/action/showPdf?pii=S2213-2600%2820%2930453-7)

From this can be seen the importance of getting the right Covid Test, asking about any test that you may have had: e.g. what type is it and how effective? Also not being afraid to ask for a different test or Antigen Test, or other available, to get 100% confirmation. After all, if the British Medical systems experts are concerned about it, then you should be too.

Are Vaccines The Answer?
The problem with vaccines is that none, as yet, have been effective in treating a "current virus". The world has seen not one, but seven coronavirus epidemics, or pandemics as they spread globally, none of these has ever had a vaccine developed for them, yet: at the time of writing (early 2021) we have no idea if any of the vaccines being developed will stop the virus, especially as it mutates fairly quickly,

usually changing before a vaccine gets out, rendering it useless. But even if they are safe; the UK Gov passed a law saying that nobody can claim damages against anyone involved in production or delivery of the vaccines; this follows the H1N1 virus - I quote a report by Dan Bloom (Mirror) stating facts about an earlier Pandemic with disastrous results -

"Ferguson H1N1 case study — Patrick Vallance — GlaxoSmithKline

At this point, I would like to go back in time to 2009 and Ferguson/Imperial College's analysis of swine flu, H1N1: they claimed this virus would take the lives of 65,000 people in the UK. In the end, 457 people died from the virus. The major difference to that and the recent Covid-19 seems to be that the latter figures were falsely reported, making deaths from it appear to be higher! That, as they say, is another story.

In response to the threat of H1N1 swine flu, Big Pharma giant GlaxoSmithKline (GSK) developed the Pandemrix vaccine, with disastrous consequences. An alleged sixty patients (new born) who suffered brain damage as a result of the vaccine were allocated £60 million in compensation by the UK Government. The victims were babies. As one report has it: "It was subsequently revealed that the vaccine, Pandemrix, can cause narcolepsy and cataplexy in about one in 16,000 people, and many more are expected to come forward with the symptoms."

Author's Considered Opinion after studying various reports from specialists in the medical system and applying logic to, mainly, UK based events.

In my considered opinion the Virus did not emanate from China in January or February 2020. It was in UK in November 2019 - confirmed by a GP, later reported on TV News after surveys and tests by various College Hospitals.

    Only a small percentage of people caught the virus and an estimated 99.01% did not. That fact was buried or hidden by Governments many times whilst they played on people's fears with psychologically designed advertisements to push the vaccines.

    Often, in the first year, various experts designated the altered PCR Test as unreliable as giving out 'False Positives'. Let us look at the logic. If you test 100 people in one area with a "dodgy" PCR Test, and just 50% read positive, then those fifty people will overfill the emergency Covid Wards in the local Hospital. If they really did not have the virus, then the chances of getting it in a packed Ward with inadequate ventilation would rise to a dangerously high proportion: but that proportion would be determined by how many of the False Positive tested who were in fact healthy enough so that their Immune System could overcome it.

For months, some NHS Doctors questioned why the Government was pushing untested and potentially dangerous vaccines when they knew that people could be successfully treated with Vitamin D or D3. In one test, carried out by one hospital, they treated one group with Vitamin D, high dose, and another with nothing. In the group who had nothing, patients died or had bad recovery rates. In the treated group, nobody died and they all recovered quickly. The Doctors asked the UK Government for an official test, on a larger scale, but they were ignored or refused! The Government instead pushed the Oxford vaccine. Neil Ferguson and others pushed the Pfizer vaccine.

In my case, November 2019, I had all the symptoms. Awoke 5 am one morning with a really horrible dry cough. At one point I could not breathe at all, so used an old Martial Arts trick for when 'winded' by a severe blow. I formed a fist and whacked myself in the Solar Plexus as hard as possible. That did the trick. I gasped and started breathing again. I had no idea it was Covid-19, but did know that it was a very aggressive virus. Living in Norfolk, UK, we are used to winter virus that often appear after a propeller engine aircraft circles between Norwich and Great Yarmouth several times during a Low Depression in weather (low cloud, pressure falling downwards!) MoD experiments have been uncovered before, so this is not imagined! This virus was dealt with by gargling with Whiskey, then doing what, traditionally, we always do with a virus, sweat it out!

It was later when I realised that I had been so busy that I forgot to take my regular supplement of Vitamin D, C, Magnesium, Selenium, etcetera. I had only taken Calcium and Zinc every few days, which, to be honest, probably helped fight it. Since then I have used a night drink of Honey & Lemon, diluted with Spring Water to clear the lungs of mucus and unwanted garbage, taken a daily Vitamin supplement and this works. My Immune System is now strong again.
I see the masks and enforced lock-downs as a possible way of making people weaker so that they have to resort to a vaccine. (End)

As a Taoist, I try to follow natural ways. This is hard to do in the West, and there has to be be times when exceptions might be considered, such as Supplements. Looking at vaccines vs diet logically though, it would seem that by taking vaccines to counter every bout of Flu (each one different from the last), or Virus, such as Covid-19, then you are bypassing the Immune System. If we do not allow the Immune System to intercept and kill virus, then the Immune system will gradually "go to sleep", so to speak. This could be very dangerous indeed!

A healthy Immune System will detect any new germs or virus, then attack it and kill it. It then "learns" from this detection and stores the ID for some time, anything from 3 to 8 months normally, sometimes longer. After this, the Immune system "forgets" the invader, but not before the recognition pattern has been passed on to the killer Lymphocytes in the body. **T-Cells** can remain actively aware of a particular viral strain for a lot longer than the Immune System, which like the vaccines, is only active for a shorter term. There are, according to some experts in epidemiology and related subjects, perhaps some longer term problems with taking too many vaccines and anti-dote drugs, creating a situation whereby the Immune System attacks itself.

The current virus and its mutated versions are quite strong, so strong that not everybody can be saved, not even after being injected with vaccines. Given the death rate, just 00.02%, or between 1 and 2 in 100, and these unfortunates having "underlying health problems (seen or unseen) already", then most people might not be so worried. The NHS of Great Britain has suggested that people who have been worst affected and/or died may also have been deficient in Vitamin D also. The UK Government has not published these facts or medical opinions though, for some odd reason. The public *should* question this, as they should with everything that Governments do "in their name".

It appears that many Governments are treating the Symptoms and not the Cause: they are looking at only artificial vaccines rather than trying to fix the main problem which is ill-health, bad diet/lifestyle and weak Immune System - metabolic syndrome. They are treating the two groups, healthy and unhealthy, the same way, but the unhealthy are those most at risk. This means that the healthier people, more able to fight any virus, are being put through unnecessary lock-downs and measures that are ruining lives and the economy. What they should be doing, according to many medical experts, is correcting the diets of the "unhealthy" and the way they think about food and exercise.

There is the choice then, big Pharma vaccines or diet and natural health. That choice is yours and yours alone.

Diet & Exercise.
Diet is extremely important in the upkeep of the human body and its many complex systems within. Having read the section on Vitamins & Minerals, you should by now have a simple understanding of just how important these are in any diet. If you have not read that section then please do so as it is for your own benefit to understand what "food" really is.

The Spanish Federation of Nutrition Societies (FESNAD) has recommended to keep the Immune System as strong as possible during Lock-downs, or any other extended indoor period. Resting and reducing stress levels are important. They do not rule out any specific foods, but say that diets based on whole grains and cereals (bread, pasta, rice), fruit and vegetables provide the best amounts of fibre (roughage) for healthy gut or intestinal motility. Choosing these fibre-rich foods helps you to avoid constipation and also promotes good digestion.

Limit or avoid processed foods (see elsewhere in this book) or processed juices (not fresh or natural) as these usually have excess sugar in. You need to drink at least one and a half litres of water, fruit juice, teas and soups a day, varying is obviously good, to maintain hydration levels.

Avoid excess snacking and maintain a regular eating regime of three meals a day: small snacks in-between if hungry mid-morning or afternoon - not in the evening (see digestive system info).

Having a routine is also good for the Mind. Try not to spend time reading about illnesses, virus outbreaks or anything else which will add to stress and anxiety. It can be beneficial to have time at home, to do those odd jobs that you have been meaning to, when you get "A round toit" or hobbies that you have meant to start/finish and never did.

Stress has a negative effect on the body: skin, lungs, breathing, blood pressure, digestion, sleep and memory. Finding something to do that is relaxing and calming is very important in maintaining better health. Women are far more prone to stress than men. Do not let imaginings become fears, stay focused on something positive, like that daily schedule.

Hobbies that are relaxing are very good: detailed model making, sewing, knitting, gardening, painting (art) or the other kind, painting and decorating. These all give you something to focus on during stressful times. Remember, Ch'ang Ming – Taoist 'Long Life' Diet – is part of the world's only Holistic system of health-care. Just because this book is about Diet, does not mean that the stomach is disconnected from the rest of the body. Exercise, the right types, is also needed.

The Food Connections?
The, shall we say, "2020 Covid-Sars-2" saw many localised outbreaks. Many of those were associated with the processing and/or consumption of dead animal flesh. In great Britain alone there were They include a chicken processing site in Anglesey, where more than 150 workers have become infected with Covid-19, and plants in Wrexham and West Yorkshire, plus Three more in Norfolk. Then there were two known outbreaks in Salad Processing plants that make pre-pack sandwiches or packets of salad: these are thought to be related to the cheap labour, often from Europe, who share crowded accommodation and sometimes car-sharing too. However, the important factor here is meat, or dead animal flesh.

Scientists have warned that a chilled climate with no sunlight can allow coronavirus to thrive in meat processing plants. In Brazil, union officials allege one-fifth of the industry's employees—about 100,000 meat plant workers—have been infected. In the US, meat-processing facilities have been linked to more than 38,500 reported cases and at least 180 deaths. Meat works made up almost half of US COVID-19 hotspots in May. They were also the major initial source of infections in Australia's June "second wave" outbreak in the state of Victoria. There have also been major outbreaks in Germany, France, Spain, Ireland, Australia, Brazil and across the US.

It is thought that because of the low temperatures it has to be stored and processed in, this allows the Covid-19 Virus the best survival chances: it is, of course, "living" on the cells within the meat; poultry, pig or bovine based. In meat-packing plants, where air speeds typically exceed 100 times that, infectious droplets and aerosols would get pushed much farther much faster. How these turbulent air conditions might affect disease transmission is harder to predict. A few medical doctors say "There has been no confirmed connection between eating meat and catching Covid" or words to that effect. Tests have not been carried out though. If the main risk is thought to be "airborne" then let us look at a couple of important factors here:

(1) The animal carcase has to be moved, often carried on the shoulder, then dumped onto a hard surface. This could create airborne droplets if the Covid virus is living within the flesh under cold conditions.

(2) Test have been carried out to see if either heat or cold would kill Covid-19 Virus. These tests have not included cooking meat or any risk of consuming said flesh, especially in part-cooked, or "rare/medium-rare" cooked meats.

I find this rather odd, as every doctor and medical scientist in the world must surely understand the other, most common risks from meats, including Salmonella, Swine Flu and Avian Flu – the latter two being types of Corona Virus too!

Ban on Ad's.
Research shows that Vegans usually weigh less than Vegetarians and meat-eaters. Experts agree that a Vegan diet can help you lose weight and maintain a healthy weight without having to worry about portion size. Therefore the risk of Obesity is greatly reduced. But what about other common diseases? It was shown that Vegans also have a lower risk of 'Type 2 Diabetes', the type usually associated with diet and lifestyle. A 2019 Harvard Medical University study of more than 300,000 people revealed that eating a Vegan diet could cut the risk of developing Type 2 Diabetes by almost a quarter. In the same year, a study of 12,000 people found that those who ate mostly plant-based foods were 32 percent less likely to die from heart disease.

In July 2020, spurred on by the so-called pandemic, the UK Government launched a new strategy in a bid to tackle the threats posed by obesity. They placed a ban "junk food" TV commercials before 9 pm (unfortunately aimed for children, not adults!) and sought to end "Buy-one-get-one-free" promotions in stores. These are all positive steps but do they really go far enough? No. The one thing they still neglect is proper education of the general public about food and diet, nutrition and health maintenance.

Simple Facts.
When you are born, your Immune System is very basic and "untrained". As soon as you begin to attend school, or play with other children, germs, virus and other predator microbes attack the body. This is when

the Immune System begins to build up its Database of attackers, so that it can become stronger. By the time we reach adulthood, the Immune System is pretty tough, but it does require upkeep. We need the right diet, exercise, oxygen or "fresh air", plus the necessary Vitamins and Minerals: as mentioned before – Vitamin D & C, Zinc, Calcium, Magnesium and they think Copper and K2 may be important too. If you do not "feed" the Immune System, then it may become weaker. Many experts also think that trying to by-pass it with vaccines may also be harmful. The old saying "Use it or lose it!" comes to mind here.

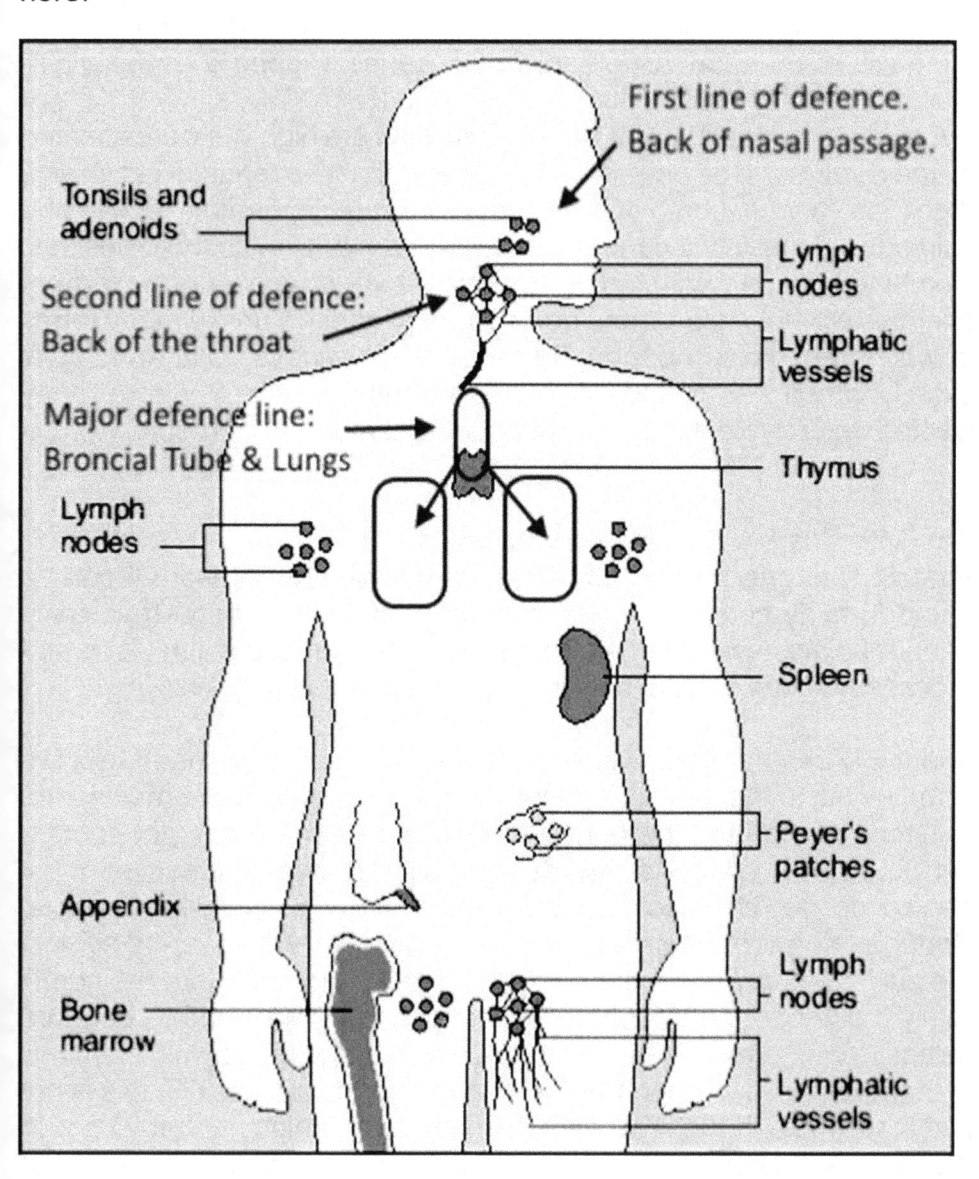

First line of defence.
Back of nasal passage.

Tonsils and adenoids

Lymph nodes

Second line of defence:
Back of the throat

Lymphatic vessels

Major defence line:
Broncial Tube & Lungs

Thymus

Lymph nodes

Spleen

Peyer's patches

Appendix

Lymph nodes

Bone marrow

Lymphatic vessels

Keeping Fit.
Exercise too is an important part of daily living. Back in the days when we were Hunter/Gatherers, we got plenty of exercise, walking, bending, twisting, plucking, digging and climbing, to name a few types of movements. Nowadays, in "modern" times, a walk from the bus-stop or car park into the local supermarket is about all the exercise many people get. Obviously not enough.

As mentioned elsewhere, exercise is not only important to keep the muscles and joints working, but it also affects digestion and, more obviously, circulation: not just of blood, but nutrients, vitamins and minerals, oxygen too. (See book in this series 'Qigong & Baduanjin')

Even exercises like T'ai Chi Ch'uan/Taijiquan are highly underestimated in their values. Not only is this a "low impact" exercise, but it aids digestion, circulation, overall body strength, mental focus and calmness, benefits the central nervous system and much more besides. Combined with a healthy diet, this simple yet so pleasurable form of exercise will help to promote good "internal health", unlike many forms of western exercise or sport. Time proven is always best, and this is exactly why it has lasted so many hundreds of years, where many western exercise crazes have died out and faded from memory.

Eat ^Vitamins & Minerals To Beat Covid!
Vitamin D is one rare but, again, a very important Vitamin. it can be found in fairly common foods, but we must bear in mind that many people's diets have changed now and for the worse: e.g. junk food and processed foods available from large chain outlets.

Vitamin D can be made within the body, but for that we need to walk, sit or lay out in the sun and get it on our whole body, or the main torso. In Great Britain, and the northern Hemisphere, we rarely get enough sun to do this, except a few days in early to mid-summer, so most people do not produce enough Vitamin D. In places like Espania, Portugal, Northern Africa, etcetera, most people try to cover-up against the sun's rays or stay in the cooler indoors areas. therefore they don't really make enough Vitamin D either. Therefore we need to be more selective with our diets. If we cannot get the right foods with vitamin D in then we can take Food Supplements instead, such as D3. this is not just that simple though, we also need minerals which our body uses in the process. These are mainly Zinc, Calcium and Magnesium, but others can also play supporting roles. Vitamin D is necessary and works with Calcium and Phosphorus to build and maintain health bones and teeth, protecting the muscles and maintaining their strength, as well as many other functions.

Evidence from around the world continues to grow that vitamin D also helps to regulate the Immune System, lower blood pressure, protect against depression, and reduce risk of type 2 diabetes, high blood pressure, and several kinds of cancer as well as possibly prevent premature deaths in otherwise quite healthy people.

Best Vitamin D Foods:
(Vegetarian or Vegan)
* Egg Yolk
* Shiitake & other Mushrooms
* Almond Milk/Soy Milk/Cows milk/Oat Milk/Yoghurt, etc.
* Almonds.
* Most "fortified" Breakfast cereals.
* Orange Juice (Fortified).
* Cheese (Dairy)/ Ricotta.
* Oatmeal.

(Cow's Milk is said to be a good source of Vitamin D as one 8 ounce glass can deliver up to 100 IU's of D or 20% of Recommended daily Allowance/DV.)

Best Zinc Foods:
Zinc is an essential mineral that plays a vital role in immune function, growth, and development. Vitamin D uses Zinc in processes.

* Baked Potatoes (with skin 6% RDA), Parsley, Zucchini and many other vegetables.

* Oatmeal.
* Fruits - Avocado, Blackberries, Cantaloupe, Raspberries, Peaches, Kiwifruits, Apricots and Blueberries.
* Tahini (a substance like peanut butter and delicious)
* Tofu (Firm)
* Lentils (Legumes), Navy, Black beans, white beans & chickpeas), Lesser amounts in Green Peas, Lima beans or cooked spinach.

* Hulled hemp seeds.
* Wild rice.
* Brazil Nuts & Cashew Nuts.
* Baking Chocolate.
* Pumpkin Seeds, Pine Nuts and Sesame Seeds.
* Soy Beans (Opting for fermented-soy dishes such as natto can also provide significant concentrations of vitamin K2 in the form of menaquinone-7.)
* Shiitake Mushrooms.
* Cereal Products that contain Wheatgerm (see Content label on Packet) & Bread.
* Most Dairy foods such as Cheese.

(Taking high doses of zinc reduces the amount of copper the body can absorb. This can lead to anaemia and weakening of the bones. So do read the %RDA advice earlier in the book and check the Daily % on the food packaging labels, which is now mandatory.)

Best Selenium & Magnesium Foods:
* Broccoli.
* Almonds, Brazil Nuts, Cashews, Pecans, Walnuts, Pine Nuts.
* Eggs
* Dark Chocolate
* Avocado Pears, Bananas, Breadfruit, Grape Juice, Guava, Tamarinds, Plantains, Papaya, Blackberries, Raspberries, Cantaloupe, Grapefruit and Dried Figs.
* Quinoa (fruit - quinoa offers 8 grams of complete protein and all nine essential amino acids — rare for non-animal protein. It also has 3.5 grams of healthy fat and 5 grams of fiber - [source-AlgaeCal.com])

Best Vitamin K Foods:
Note: anyone using Warfarin must *not* binge on high K foods as this could provoke harmful results! Intake should be measured and steady, under advice.

* Most of the leafy green vegetables contain Vitamin K.
* Most of the nuts, beans, fruits, Tofu and cereals listed above.
* Algae products - check out what is available in your area and what the contents are.

As you can see, this starts to create a pattern of foods that can form part of a healthy breakfast, lunch and dinner. There are many other foods which contain varying amounts of the above Vitamins/Minerals.

Here I have just started you off with a few suggestions that may be found world-wide. Knowing what you need to look for now, reading labels on food packs is an easy way forward and also help you to learn about your diet.

Summary:
Humans have always been prone to virus, just as other animals have. Most other animals eat a normal diet, foods which their body need. Humans can easily be fooled into thinking that anything processed, wrapped and sold as "food", therefore must be food. It is not! Hopefully you will have taken on board the facts and comments about processed foods, like White Sugar: made from Beet, a root vegetable, and not 'natural' but *refined*. Chocolate, sweets, all artificial foodstuffs, if consumed regularly, especially in place of a wholesome meal, WILL CAUSE HEALTH PROBLEMS, as will a build-up of Toxins, or other agents that are not good fro the body.

End of special needs section, for now!

A SENSIBLE DIET
What Is It Today?

Supermarkets tend to be the norm now. The bigger the chain the more hope that you may have of finding something decent to eat in there. The lesser known supermarket chains may offer pure, unashamed rubbish disguised thinly as foods by using chemicals These are normally processed, non-organic, genetically modified (GM) and laden with additives, colours and flavours. So where do we get what we need?

Standardisation dictates most food businesses, especially in the European Union. A great pity. The petty bureaucrats are once again defacing and defiling our lives at the same time as taking away freedom of choice and the choices themselves, (diversity). The only thing which replaces that diversity nowadays are a few pre-prepared dishes from the likes of the common supermarkets which are plonked into little plastic dishes, covered in plastic film and are ready to "nuke" in the microwave. These are usually, like all the other substances, laced with additives, colourings and preservatives. Even "alternative" foods, such as organic farm produce, are possibly subject to problems:

Because of distribution it may take longer to reach stores (therefore lose goodness, vitamins begin to decay, et cetera).
It is thought that some organic produce may be sprayed with pesticide or other chemicals whilst in the grain silo or on the barn floor.

Organic produce is limited to few products in most areas.

There are a few food chains working on this problem and trying to bring us a more fresh and unadulterated line or selection of organic foods. We also have to thank the Iceland chain for starting the pressure against GM foods. So, between the big four (in UK) we may find some GM free, organic produce. Big deal. We may also find some small local shops which sell organic produce too, these shops may not offer the freshest of produce, like vegetables, but are worth supporting for many other things, like local honey.

Once you have done your scouting there is no reason in the world why you should not be able to buy and eat tasty, wholesome, organic foods that are going to make you feel and look better. Using organic brown rice (short grain) as a staple, along with some wholemeal bread (as long as you are not allergic to wheat!) and a few variants, can make for some pretty satisfying dishes. So it is possible to eat a healthy diet nowadays, and getting better by the year, so really try and persevere.

Note: If you have time you can even make your own preserves, beer or wine, all from what Mother Nature provides, free and local. At the time of update, it is becoming more widely thought that one or two beers daily can help reduce the chance of Heart attack or Strokes.

The sole purpose of this book is to *educate* you, the reader, so that you may deduce for yourself what might be good, bad or indifferent for your health. Use the reference tables (Five Elements and Yin/Yang) and the references to what foods are, do for you or to you, vitamins and minerals, 'Foods With Attitude', and then start to examine your diet: not forgetting the advice to carefully 'List and Lose', one thing at a time!

SAMPLE DIET MENU

Be warned, this section is not intended for you to follow to the letter, but just as an example of what a day's balanced diet *might* look like for someone experienced.

Please remember that is is NOT a diet to follow, just an example of how you might try to balance foods and drinks in a day. The main objective for you is to *change*. Then study more, discover more, learn and apply using common sense and knowledge.

Practical Example of Balanced Daily Diet:

Breakfast (6-7 am)
Porridge Oats or Wholemeal Toast+   Oats or Grain Cereal.
 Mixed Grain & Dry Fruit Fresh Fruit as a follower, not 'main'.

Lunch (11am-1pm)

Wholemeal Pasta & veg.	Salad/Beans/Nuts.
Veg. Casserole/Curried	Vegetables. Baked Potato & veg.
Veg. Stew/Roast.	Fruit Salad/Legumes.
Oatcakes/Cereals	Dried Fruit/Pot.Sal*

Dinner (5-7 pm)
Fruit. Sweet & Sour Veg. Fruit Salad/Nuts. (No Carb's in the evening as the metabolism slows down. Protein based.)

Drinks: Dandelion Coffee, Herb Tea[1], Fruit Juice or 'Smoothie', water.

Occasional: Fruit, dried fruit (winter), nuts (winter), cereal bars/biscuits (low sugar).

*Potato Salad: placed here only for practicality in modern western living. Potatoes are Yin, but also a source of 'quick energy' complex carbohydrates, which if you are going out in the evening or training should 'burn off' rather than settle and cause fatty deposits from unspent energy.

 ** Rice is best if short grain whole.

These are just loose examples to give you ideas and can be added to or varied according to (a) what is available in your area where you work, (b) what you have available at home. Bearing in mind that we should have the proverbial Five Vegetables and Three Fruit portions per day, then we can add what else we need. In this day and age, with quick chilled and ready prepared foods, we can of course take a few short cuts in our busy lives: use fruit smoothies, pre-packed meals (not processed) from the supermarket, etcetera. Sometimes we have no choice but to do these things.

---

[1] In some other forms of Buddhism meat is eaten, strangely enough. This may be due to lack of vegetables and fruit (odd as it takes much vegetation to rear an animal!) or, more likely, a personal unwillingness or lack of self-will to give it up.

If you fancy a traditional style 'Sunday lunch' you can have it, but even healthier. You can use vegetable protein pieces instead of meats, vegetarian gravy (boosted with mushrooms and onions, maybe some garlic), roast potatoes, vegetables and even Yorkshire puddings. Delicious!

Once in a while, if I have a long or hard day of work or physical training such as a weekend workshop, a vegetarian 'fry up' is called upon. This consists of wholemeal toast, beans, tomato, egg and perhaps hash browns all done in a light olive oil. It may not be "ideal" Zhangming but when you are staying at a B&B and choices are limited, then you have top make do. There are enough complex carbohydrates to create energy in abundance, a bit of fruit and a cereal bar during the lunch-break keeps me going until dinnertime.

The Five Flavours
Revisit the Five Elements table. Here you will see how the Chinese have associated the five flavours with five elements of health. We should have a mixture of these types of food in our daily or weekly diet: e.g. Sweet, Bitter, Pungent, Salty & Sour, to maintain a 'balanced' diet alongside the fruit and vegetables.

Dietetics, Herbs, Drugs or What?

When illness comes knocking, and it does for 99.9% of us, then you have to do several things. Firstly, sit back and take stock; what are the symptoms? Next you have to realise from the symptoms what it is you have been doing wrong, and then stop it. Following this is the remedy. All remedies *should be* "horses for courses" as we say. I have italicised "should be" as many people tend to stick with one health practitioner and go to a chiropractor for an upset stomach, for example. This may sound silly, but I hear of such things all the time. Some are more subtle, like the woman who complained of lower back pains. This came on after the arrival of a new baby to her daughter-in-law, over which she fussed and drooled, of course; who wouldn't! After asking her a couple of questions and sensing some "Ah Shi!" points on her bio-energy (Ch'i) Meridians, I suggested that she went to see a good Shiatsu Massage practitioner. She almost adamantly refused and said that she would go see her chiropractor as she always did. As they say, you can lead a horse to water, but you can't make it drink. If only people would take some good advice from those who are more experienced in these matters. Although I do not know everything, I have been dealing with such problems for thirty-five years (up to 2002 and have a reasonably sound lay knowledge of what's what in the imbalances and illnesses world. Thus I am able to suggest the right practitioner for the dis-ease.

Dietetics

This is the art of food and balance. Although a few Western Orthodox (e.g. hospital) dieticians still recommend things such as animal liver or read meat (which generally make a positive difference to the people they are treating), I feel strongly, given my studies and research, that these should not be included in a healthy diet and can cause many other problems, too many to list here. The Taoists have, over many hundreds of years, experimented and gathered information about different types of food and what they can and will do to both humans and animals. This research dates back and precedes modern western research, which often seems contradictory or even uncertain. One only has to look at most modern food scientists and measure their health, fitness and life-span, then compare that with traditional Taoists who have been known to live to 100 years or even 180 years where external pollutants are not a worrying factor. I know where I feel better off!

Dietetics should be the art of balancing your diet so that the food and drink you intake rids you of pathogens, and toxins, as well as giving you strength (energy and body building materials), vitality and better health. Adjusting your diet to suit what you do (work, leisure or exercise), your state of health, or your environment (eat local produce as much as possible) is essential for better health and a longer, happier life.

Using this book as a guide to food and diet should be easy, especially if you have been advised by a 'professional' and are not at all sure of what she or he has told you to eat. Now you can check it for yourself. Western Orthodox dietetics often does not take into account chemicals and chemical reactions, additives, toxins, hormones and injections or growth inducers in animals for the food chain, and many other factors that are unnatural and therefore harmful. We even see ignorant doctors on television advocating women to eat more red meat: when it has been scientifically proven to be a cancer causative?[1] Doctors should not advise on matters they do not understand or have not specialised in. There may be many who criticise me for writing this book by saying,

---

[1] If the body lacks the supportive elements then pathogens (disease forming situations) set in.

"he's not a doctor!" No I am not, and I don't profess to be, but what I *am* is a Chinese Traditional Health and Fitness practitioner and as such have studied my subjects for many years: more years than it takes to become a family GP/doctor. I would never advise anything which I would not do myself or that I have not researched or looked deeply into. Moreover, myself and many other living and known Taoists are or have been living proof of the Tai Chi Diet and its effectiveness at prolonging life and extending good health.

Food of the improper kind causes most illnesses and the right food can also cure most illnesses; unlike drugs which normally cover the symptoms of one illness whilst setting up side-effects that are equally bad or worse! The improper kind of foods are outlined in this book, so there is no point in going over that ground twice, so to speak. By studying this book and learning which foods are good for you and which are bad you can change your health. In fact you can change your life.

Herbs
When I studied Herbalism there was little access to information about Chinese Herbalism and the Oriental herbs that it uses. This was not an unhappy choice for me though as Western Herbalism is rich in simple remedies and we who live in the West (Europe, UK and USA) have an abundance of our 'local' herbs, many growing wild all around us. This reminds me of the story of how "caddies" (catty, pronounced "caddy", being roughly the Chinese equivalent of 1lb in English weight) of Chinese Tea came to be sold in England, or exchanged for our herbs:

A Chinese merchant seaman arrived in London in the era when tea was scarce and expensive. He noticed that the "trendies" of the time were raving about tea, or "Cha" to give it its Chinese name. He also noticed that sage was growing wild around the commons and countryside. Being shrewd, as most Chinese are, he offered a trader "one Catty of tea for two Catties (pronounced 'caddies') of that useless wild herb". The trader, who thought that the Chinese man was mad, said yes very quickly. He wondered why the Chinese man would want the odd weed that no one else wanted. The deal was struck. The Chinese man became a big trader in his own right and brought half a ship's hold of tea over. He took a hold full of sage back in return.

The English trader was in his element. He made plenty of money. The Chinese trader made even more. You see the Chinese believe that sage is the best tea for health and long life, hence the name that we know it by, "sage" (wise person or wisdom). Even though the Chinese may not have known about carcinogens (potentially harmful element of the tea leaf) they certainly knew that sage was much better for you!

Herbs are very natural and very powerful. They can bolster your immune system, help you recover from illness, make you urinate more, or less, they can help you sleep, gain a better appetite, lose weight, energise your weary body, rest or become more calm and many more things besides. You should only use herbs when necessary and when prescribed and prepared by someone who knows what they are doing; Never go out and pick herbs, berries or mushrooms for that matter, if you are not 100% sure of what you are doing!

Chinese herbalists are in every city nowadays in the UK. Practice caution and seek first hand inspection of their credentials, in English, not Chinese! I say this because I have seen one local young Chinese woman in a bookshop, using books as a reference for symptoms and apparently seeking an answer to some illness or imbalance that she did not understand. Also, a friend who has trained in acupuncture and had much experience in Chinese herbs has told me that some herbs can be very toxic. Nowadays they are grown or picked in large quantities to supply the world's burgeoning market, so they may not be picked at the right time and this may cause certain chemical or toxic reactions when prepared in a mixture. This is what I have been told. At another time I sought a small clinic where I could rent a couch or massage room for interviewing people who come to me with health problems. I visited a small office space in a shared building where two English girls dealt in Chinese herbs. One said that she was qualified. During a conversation about diagnostics it became apparent they did not use comprehensive methods. They would ask a person what was wrong and then look up the symptoms and treat the client. From my humble experience of TCM it is my understanding that any Traditional Chinese Medicine practitioner, be it herbs, acupuncture or Tui Na, would spend at least one hour interviewing the client on the first occasion and determine facts about diet, lifestyle and any other medications being taken; as obviously mixing drugs and herbs could be drastic, or deadly! The two girls were not familiar with my reasoning, so I left them with a complete diet and lifestyle questionnaire that I had devised for the purpose. Hopefully they will have amended their approach.

The simple moral of these stories is? Please go to established herbalists with recognised qualifications. I do not wish to rule out those people who are not formally trained, especially as I have learned much in that mode and it would be hypocritical to do so. A simple rule of thumb is to gauge the quality of the practitioner by the amount of time they spend asking questions and in diagnostics, as the real cause of your illness or disease must be determined and all roads explored.

Drugs

I personally think that orthodox medicine has lost its way and has buried its head in the sand for far too long. Doctors and therapists are bound by too many Pharmaceutical or other principles that are restricting and narrow. Whilst it is not possible to give someone free reign to use anything or act in a random manner without knowledge, it would make more sense if the tried and true were used also, or instead of. Orthodox medicine has been far too slow to recognise treatments like acupuncture, but even then, when it apparently has, some traditionally trained acupuncturists have expressed horror at the short length of time that orthodox acupuncturists have spent in training. They also criticise the lack of diagnostics and use of "general points" without full diagnostics. Drugs and surgery are the rule of orthodox practitioners and as many people know, drugs kill. Recently a fact was released in medical journals that over 2,000 people in the UK die each year as a result of prescribed painkillers. How many more die as a result of those bought over the counter I wonder?

I once received a fax for a neighbour who was involved in the drugs industry (I used to refer to him as a "Drug Peddler"!). The fax was from someone who had performed a talk at a surgery in front of many local GP's. The meeting's Minutes told a complete horror story. Amongst many drug issues on it were casual facts that the manufacturers (a very big name) had stopped producing some drugs, usually prescribed for depression, anxiety or pain, or mixtures of these, as they had been successful in killing many patients! These were to be replaced with new drugs; no doubt to be used on even more guinea pigs... sorry, I mean patients!

Supplements

Scientific tests and experiments around the world have concluded that the inclusion of regular (recommended daily doses: RDA) of the following minerals in your daily diet will, amongst other things:

- lessen risk of most common cancers and tumours
- reduce infertility and increase sperm count and sexual libido
- reduce risk of cataracts, growth impairment, heart disease and infections (immunity), etc.
- reduce acne, mental illness & depression, etc., poor hair growth, slow healing, poor growth in children, age spots, loss of muscle tone, osteoporosis, help the activation an process of many hormones, decrease nervousness, rashes,etc.
- Help impaired taste, smell, some cases of gum disease, and many more.

What are these fantastic but often missed minerals? Simple and available from all good health shops, they are calcium, magnesium, zinc and selenium. Especially if you are a man, in later life[1], and lacking a good and healthy sex life, then these come highly recommended, but you will need a healthy woman who will appreciate the benefits, so look after her diet too!

Note: Always check your daily intake of vitamins and supplements against the RDA so that you do not overdose! See Chapter on Vitamins in this book.)

---

[1] Source of information - The Nutritional Health Bible by Linda Lazarides.

COMPLIMENTARY EXERCISES

There is absolutely no excuse for not taking part in some form of exercise if you have use of your legs or arms. Even those confined to a bed for some period of time need exercise and can do something, like the adapted Form of Pa T'uan Chin (Baduanjin), for example, a beautiful and gentle set of stretching and breathing exercises which not only work the physical aspects of the body, externally and internally, but help open the energy channels and heal, balance and refresh too.

There are many, many forms of exercise that derive from China. If you walk through virtually any Chinese street in the early morning or still of the evening then you are bound to see hundreds of people doing hundreds of different exercises. Whilst it may not be possible to nip down to your local park in Six Mile Bottom, Bognor Regis or even Norwich and see such sights there may well be an instructor of Chinese health and fitness regimes at a hall somewhere near you.

For the medical fraternity especially, you should look at Dr Paul Lam's website, www.TaiChiForArthritis.com, for here you will find interesting links to research carried out on the medical benefits of Taijiquan. When I first started this book Taijiquan's health benefits were virtually unknown in the West, now it has enjoyed a boom worldwide and many medical establishments are waking up to the possibilities of both curative and preventative properties of a gentle form of Taijiquan, Tai Chi for Health. Some establishments are already using or enquiring about our wonderful Tiandidao Baduanjin (Eight Strands of Silk Brocade) exercise set which has been brought up to date for medical safety. This has wonderful remedial and preventative properties.

Internet Connections
If you are one of the many who has access to the Internet then finding someone may be fairly easy. Try some of these UK URL's (Uniform resource Location), or website addresses:

www.TTTkungfu.com
(The author's school's website & BBS) Find Links to National Instructors. www.AMAA.org.uk
(Association for all Martial Arts Instructors)

The above links are enough to get you started. Failing all that, or if you are not connected, you can try to get information at your local Library. UK libraries have what they call an ICON database. This can have many contacts in it for all sorts of recreational activities. You may also find that, like our new Forum Library in Norwich, they have Internet connected computer terminals that you can use for free, so you could check out those websites above after all.

There must be something out there which takes your fancy, be it walking, jogging, joining a fitness club, Taiji, Qigong, Gongfu, get a good Personal Trainer or play Badminton, do some Yoga or some other form of exercise. Whatever you actively do it is far, far better than sitting on your bum and being a so-called 'couch potato'. So, change your diet and make a fresh start. However, always seek advice on exercise first and if you are unsure about your ability to exercise then consult your GP or therapist first.

Exercise is essential for a healthy body, heart, lungs, muscles and heart; and includes circulation, nervous system and other beneficial side-effects as well as a making the mind more positive and the brain better oxygenated and therefore more efficient; this also helps sleep, rest and repair as well as helping keep the digestive and circulatory systems functioning well. Starting exercise need not be a shock to the system. In fact it should not be allowed to be. Always start slowly and gently. Then, like everything else, you can slowly pick up speed and pace. It is like starting your new diet, "list and lose". Begin by walking more, then take the stairs instead of the lift. If your heart is healthy and you have no knee or back problems, try to walk fast enough for half-an-hour each day to raise your heart rate. This should strengthen the heart and help burn off excess fat; but you must remember to eat healthy foods and more complex carbohydrates as these will give you more energy as well as help you build stronger muscles.

Starting off with some gentle Ch'i Kung (Qigong) or T'ai Chi Ch'uan (Taiji Quan) can work wonders. Even those who have arthritis or diabetes can benefit, thanks to Dr. Paul Lam, a Chinese Physician who resides in Australia. He has developed easy to learn and perform Taiji and Qigong sets which are targeted at these illnesses, based on traditional Chinese Taiji or Qigong but with cooperation and advice from some of the leading specialists in arthritis or diabetes medical fields.

So there you are. A complete new lifestyle. What are you waiting for? Start planning a better future today. List and lose!

The grass *really* is greener on the other side of the hill.

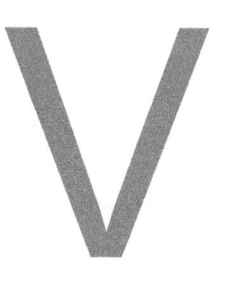

V

End Note:

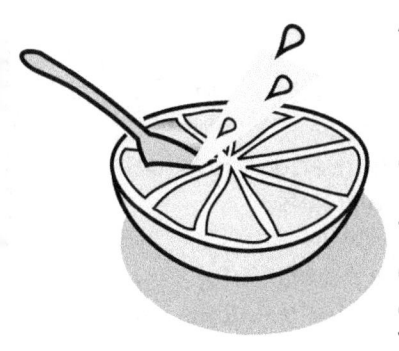

Alright, who was taking it all in?

Somewhere, not so far back was a mention of having a Honey & Lemon drink on the bedside table.

Those of you who are very observant will of course associate Honey & lemon, in one form or another, with Cold & Flu Treatments, including over-the-counter medicines. This age old recipe has been used by the pharmaceutical companies and most people will instantly grab a packet of such drugs off the shelf. But, this wonder of Nature is more than just something to ease a sore throat or subdue a cough. Honey is a natural healer and antibiotic, as well as having antiseptic properties if used on wounds! Lemon juice has some very astringent properties and will act on mucus and harmful deposits in the lungs and trachea, causing you to cough and expel them in the morning. No drugs. No known harmful side-effects and a great anti-virus aid as well as helping Lung Healer tool.

The Author's Background

RELATED QUALIFICATIONS:
Over 65 Years Training & Study in Martial Arts, Psychology, Philosophy & Related Subjects*, Herbalism, Yoga, etc.
Over 32 Years* as a Teacher (*as of 2021) and over 3,000 students.

Chief Instructor, Founder & Developer of T'ien Ti Tao P'ai or Way of Heaven & Earth School: Developed complete, holistic system over 34 plus years;
Accepted by ICKF China as "Genuine Traditional Chinese Arts" 1987.

Nominated 'Professor' of Chinese & Taoist Arts (2001).
Awarded Master of Arts, (M.A.) (c.1998).
Awarded B.N.M.A.A., Honours. (for 'Development of Kung-fu in UK').

Awarded 'Outstanding Achievements in Martial Arts' (USA Black Belt Society 1986)
Qualified Level 1 & 2 Instructor of TCA (Dr. Paul Lam)
Qualified MAGNVQ 2 Sports Coaching; equiv' UKi Standard MA

Practical Taoist Philosophy (still studying)
Teacher of Unified Tao (Wudang) System: Taoist Kung-fu & Taijiquan, Staff, Spear, Dao, Jian, Twin Dagggers, Walking Stick/Brolly, Bang & Rule, Tai Chi for Health, Baduanjin, etcetera.
Qualified Taoist K'ai Men Yoga (Li/Lee Family Arts)
Qualified Taoist Ch'ang Ming Diet (Li/Lee Family Arts)
Qualified Ch'i Kung Energy Training (Li/Lee Family Arts)
Qualified Taoist diagnostics, health & healing Arts (Li/Lee Family Arts).

Studied Kempo and other Oriental systems 1960's to 1970's.
Studied Yoga, Meditations, Western Herbalism.

Main Posts Held:
Principal Executive Officer of Ability Martial Arts Association (AMAA) UK.

East Anglian T'ai Chi for Arthritis Instructor: Dr. Paul Lam Programme.

Lecturer for Norfolk Probation Services.
Schools self-defence Instructor (Norfolk).

Former Posts Held:
East Anglian Ambassador for Kuoshu (B.K.P.A./I.C.K.F., R.o.China); also Judge and UK Events Official (BKPA/ICKF-UK & AMA).
Norfolk Representative and Events Organiser for Amateur Martial Association, UK.

Head Coach – British Association for Chinese Arts.

Dietary & Health Advisor to Fitness Professional .co.uk

Schools Self-defence Program (Post Curriculum)

Women's Specific Self-defence Programme.

Creator of 'Staff Jousting' Sport.

Author of several books including this series of Taoist Arts Books seeking to preserve traditional knowledge that is still valid in modern society.

BIBLIOGRAPHY of REFERENCE

The Tao of Long Life: The Chinese Art of Chang Ming
  by Clifford Chee Soo
    ISBN: 0-86033-068-0
    Gordon & Cremonesi

Chinese Yoga – The Chinese Art of Kai Men
  by Professor Chee Soo
    ISBN: 0-86033-033-2
    Gordon & Cremonesi

Body Wisdom
  by Jennifer Harper
    ISBN: 0-7225-3368-3   Thorsons

Macrobiotics
  by Nyoiti Sakurazawa
    (ISBN ?)
    Tandem

The Nutritional Health Bible
  by Linda Lazarides
    ISBN: 0-7225-3424-8   Thorsons

The Yellow Emperor's Classic of Internal Medicine
  by Ilza Veith
    ISBN: 0520-02158-4   University California

Chinese Medicine – The Web That Has No Weaver
  by Ted J.Kaptchuk
    ISBN: 0-09-153231-0
    Rider

Collins Gem – Natural and Artificial Food Additives.
  By Collins
    ISBN: 0-00-458992-0

Author's own books in this Taoist Arts series:
(to 2021)

Practical Philosophy of Tao
for schools and individuals ISBN: 9780954293208

Qigong & Baduanjin
Complete Sets of Eight Strands of Silk Brocade.
ISBN: 9780954293222

T'ai Chi Ch'uan – The Wellspring Source Book.
Comprehensive coverage of history, development, philosophy behind it, and more.
ISBN: 9780954293253

UK NHS Website - Various references.

Harvard Medical University - Various references and studies.

Specialist Food or Diet Organisations.

CPSIA information can be obtained
at www.ICGtesting.com
Printed in the USA
BVHW041344020821
613407BV00011B/410